# THE GREATEST
# COLLEGE
# HEALTH
# GUIDE
## YOU NEVER KNEW
## YOU NEEDED

# THE GREATEST
# COLLEGE
# HEALTH
# GUIDE
## YOU NEVER KNEW
## YOU NEEDED

**How to Manage Food, Booze, Stress, Sex, Sleep, and Exercise on Campus**

JILL AND DAVE HENRY

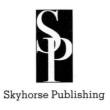

Skyhorse Publishing

Skyhorse Publishing books may be purchased in bulk at special discounts for sales promotion, corporate gifts, fund-raising, or educational purposes. Special editions can also be created to specifications. For details, contact the Special Sales Department, Skyhorse Publishing, 307 West 36th Street, 11th Floor, New York, NY 10018 or info@skyhorsepublishing.com.

Skyhorse® and Skyhorse Publishing® are registered trademarks of Skyhorse Publishing, Inc.®, a Delaware corporation.

Visit our website at www.skyhorsepublishing.com.

10 9 8 7 6 5 4 3 2 1

Library of Congress Cataloging-in-Publication Data is available on file.

Cover design by Daniel Brount

Print ISBN: 978-1-5107-5909-1
Ebook ISBN: 978-1-5107-5910-7

Printed in China

*To the team.*

# CONTENTS

# CHAPTER 1

# ORIENTATION

## PART 1: DAVE

**One month after winter break, I found the first evidence of change in a picture my friend pulled up from the night before.** I can't recall the exact theme of the party, but I was wearing a red bandana, covered in face paint, and shirtlessly drinking out of a giant glass boot. I looked . . . *different.* Swollen. My entire torso was enormous. It appeared as though I'd swallowed a barrel, but not in a barrel-chested or "that guy's built like a brick shithouse" kind of way. It looked like I'd swallowed an *inflatable* barrel that people would use as a pool toy. And I was so pale! Really pale. If not for my beet-red face, I had the milky complexion of a cadaver or an albino lab rat kept in a basement. After growing up in California, one semester in Iowa had turned my body into a ghostly couch cushion. I stared at that picture in astonishment, thinking, *Why didn't anybody tell me that I look like this?*

I had no idea how to take care of myself when I got to college. Most people don't. That's probably because once you're away from your parents and on your own for the first time, the notion that you'd be prepared to set some ground rules for yourself is absolutely ridiculous. In high school, it's easy to eat the food that's in your fridge or the meal that's made for you. It's easy to turn down booze when you know you'll get grounded if you're caught, or to get enough sleep when there's a knock on your door if the lights aren't out by midnight. All that changes when you're dropped off on campus and left to fend for yourself. It's the beginning of independence, and it is incredible, but it also increases the chances that you're going to accidentally adopt some habits that are *really* bad for your health. That's certainly what happened to me.

I religiously stayed up late, drank four nights a week, and regularly ate a large pizza around midnight. The dining hall entrées typically tasted like garbage and looked as if the entire plate had once been a canned good, so I survived on burgers. Often two or three of them, accompanied by an additional *plate* full of fries. After my meat feast, I'd hit the soft-serve machine, getting seconds before leaving simply because it was there. It's no wonder why six months straight of gluttonous chaos made me look like *Moby Dick* just in time for spring break.

From a health standpoint, the college environment is comically designed for you to fail. Want to have a few beers on a Tuesday? No problem! You'll definitely find someone on your floor to join. Want to bail on exercise and take an afternoon nap? Great idea, I love naps. If you want to play video games until four in the morning, that's okay too. Your RA isn't going to tell you to go to bed. And if you're too tired to go to class in the morning, you *can* skip it. Seriously. There's little chance your professor is going to check in. While some people seem to be able to balance the stress of schoolwork, social life, and cruise-ship-buffet-style eating while living on vampire hours, I found the vast majority of my peers in the deep end with me, struggling to swim. What's strange is that I hadn't noticed the patterns I was picking up or the toll they were taking on my physical and mental health. I'd been led to believe that was just how everybody lived, because, frankly, it sort of is.

The "Freshman 15" is widely talked about, and chances are good that you know at least one person who came home for Thanksgiving break looking a little *different* than when they left in September. Nearly 25 percent of college freshmen gain ten pounds in their first semester alone.[1] I gained twelve. But while an increase (or decrease) in weight might be the most obvious repercussion of living like an animal on campus, that's only the tip of the iceberg—just one possible side effect of being overwhelmed by too much *everything*. Access to temptation coupled with a lack of structure creates a perfect storm, which brings about an increased risk of many other health concerns, such as chronic stress, severe sleep deprivation, anxiety, depression, alcohol abuse, eating disorders, and suicide. College isn't easy. And the simple prob-lem at the heart of most struggles for the millions of students who enter every year? A lack of knowledge about how to effectively take care of themselves.[2]

I'd never thought about any of this until I headed back to high school, but not in a *Billy Madison* kind of way. I started coaching football part-time to bring more balance and meaning to my work life and was instantly rewarded with all the good feelings that come from helping people work hard and reach their goals. As the graduating classes moved on to colleges across the country, I'd inevitably hear stories that sounded similar to my own when I checked in with former players. They were eating like shit, pulling all-nighters, and had completely given up on exercise. My typical response was to listen, reply with my own horror story, and end with the sentiment, "Well, you know what they say: everyone shits their pants in college." Connecting with alums over the challenges of campus life was an unexpectedly entertaining part of the job, but I never really knew how to help them better navi-gate the pitfalls they were facing. The answers wouldn't become apparent until years after I met my wife.

Jill is the girls' cross-country coach and a math teacher at that same high school. Our first few encounters felt like an awkward teenager rom-com but applied to adults in PE clothes. Eventually, the head football coach at the time, a fully tattooed former MMA fighter, came up to me at practice and let me know that I had a "secret admirer." His face was a mix of confusion and delight when he shared that she had referred to me as a "stone-cold fox" after confirming with him that I was single.

I've never met anyone like Jill. She's incredibly disciplined and responsible but has a surprisingly foul mouth and an endearingly immature sense of humor. She will find a way to turn anything into a game, but mostly because she enjoys shit-talking anyone who can handle it. She grew up in New England, and after meeting her family, I came to understand that that's kind of a thing there. My brother aptly described her once as a cartoon character due to her endless supply of energy and use of sound effects, which she applies to everyday actions like tying her shoes or unloading groceries.

We've been teammates since the beginning of our relationship. Health was a priority for both of us before we met because we'd learned the hard way that it's impossible to feel good without taking care of yourself. We each struggled with health for the first time while in college, and there we were, years later, still trying to master good habits. It felt natural to continue those efforts together. For years, we read books and articles and played around with different routines and structures, noting what seemed to make a difference and what was just a headache. We often talked about this trial and error with our athletes. While the failures made for better stories, the successes, along with research, helped broaden our understanding of what was needed to kick ass in every area. We never thought we'd really do anything with what we'd learned until one of Jill's senior runners asked her after the last race of the season, "Coach, how do I *not* get fat in college?"

## PART 2: JILL

**As a cross-country coach, I take great pride in assigning clever names to our team workouts.** *Horseshoe of Death. Pyramid of Pain. Shovel of Doom.* The more difficult the workout, the more whimsical the title. *The Ice Cream Cone Run.* You might think that one sounds awesome. My team certainly did, until I explained that the objective was to run up a mountain on a hot day without melting. The expectation versus the delivered product was a contrast that delighted me. My runners didn't think it was funny.

Though I sometimes play the hard-ass when we're all together, I care deeply about my athletes. Working with them is about more than just training. In cross-country, we spend runs engaging with one another. Coaches and athletes conversing freely, sharing about the ups and downs of our days, airing frustrations and concerns, having a laugh, or swapping advice. Over the course of each season, we become a family, and the roads and trails become our proverbial dinner table. By the time my runners graduate, I've formed meaningful relationships with many of them. There's a mutual trust and shared respect that is a direct result of spending four years working *together*. I run each of those horrifying workouts with my athletes, by their side, encouraging them to push through the pain every step of the way. The workouts destroy me too, but sharing those experiences with my girls is one of the best parts of my job. Witnessing them realize how capable they are is a privilege. They not only learn how to work hard, they develop confidence in themselves. They discover that they're strong enough to come out on top when shit hits the fan. It took me a long time to learn those lessons, and I mostly got there alone. So while it's important to me to foster an environment that encourages toughness, it's more important to create a space where vulnerability is seen as a strength, support is given freely, and growth is nurtured, not forced.

When my runner asked me, "How do I not get fat in college?" she wasn't joking. She was scared. She didn't even know where she'd be going to school yet, but the idea of managing her health alone had brought her close to tears. I promised to do whatever I could to help. She wanted to know how to stay healthy once she was on campus, which put her one significant step ahead of where I'd been at her age. I didn't know how to take care of myself before I got to college and had no idea at the time that I even needed to. Neither did Dave.

He was an all-state quarterback in high school who went on to play not one but two college sports. He's still an athletic machine when he wants to be. Just recently, on a day where he was particularly fired up, one of his coworkers overheard Dave muttering to himself, "I think I could run through a wall right now." Dave instead decided to run up a nearby *mountain* with the goal of making it back before the end of his lunch break. If it wasn't for his inability to resist burritos and beer and his firm resistance to going to bed before midnight, he might have made it through college (and his twenties) with his health unscathed.

As he said earlier, we met while coaching. By then, he had figured out how to take care of himself and was invested in getting even better at it. What he hadn't figured out was that asking someone (*me*) out on a first date after practice while within earshot of fifty or so high school students was insane. We both endured a chorus of *oohs* and *awws* as we clumsily exchanged numbers. I was then immediately subjected to an onslaught of dating advice from my runners: *Don't make him do math problems. Don't challenge him to a push-up contest. Oh! And don't talk in your man voice—it's creepy.* I won't say they are the reason we went on a second date, but I will admit that it was probably time to scrap the line I'd been using at bars ("solve this equation and you'll have my number").

Although we figured out how to function like adults before meeting each other, we both screwed up mightily in college with our mental and physical health. My own bumpy ride is what inspired me to start teaching my athletes how to take care of themselves. That information is particularly useful in cross-country, where the only weapon you can bring to battle is your body. If you treat it like garbage, that's how you'll perform. So, I spend time every summer teaching the wellness basics. My runners learn about nutrition because you can't fuel workouts on fries and soda. They learn about sleep because you can't get stronger if you never rest. They learn about stress management because you can't do *anything* well if you are always over-whelmed. My immediate goal was that the knowledge would help them excel as runners, but my ultimate hope was that after four years of sticking to healthy rou-tines, they would feel prepared to take care of themselves even after high school sports were over. Unfortunately, they didn't. They already knew what I hadn't been even remotely aware of at their age: college would be different, and many of their current good habits wouldn't survive the transition.

As much as he loved it, Dave's crazy work schedule ultimately forced him to step away from coaching football a few years after we got married. However, he filled that void by working with my team whenever he could. When my runner asked for help, it was no surprise that Dave wanted to work with me to provide the solution. That said, we definitely never set out to write a book. Our initial plan was to prepare a packet of workouts and meal suggestions for the seniors in hopes that some basic guidance would be enough to help them avoid making the mistakes we had. But at some point we realized that, based on our own experience, learning how to take care of yourself is an *enormous* undertaking that can't be condensed into a tiny guide. We expressed that sentiment to the seniors at a postseason team brunch, saying, "We're sorry we don't have something for you yet, but there's so much content to cover that we could write a book!" We will both never forget the moment that one of them looked at us and said, with complete sincerity, "You should."

After considering that seemingly outlandish suggestion for weeks, we high-fived like idiots and decided to go for it. We spent a year doing countless hours of research on food, booze, exercise, stress, and sleep. We sent out hundreds of anonymous surveys to college students. We rehashed the details of our own failures, and then put them on paper for the first time. Oh, in the middle of all of that, we had a baby!

Despite wanting to help you avoid the same traps we fell into, we are firm believers that it's impossible to be perfect with your health. It's also unnecessary. Yes, taking care of yourself requires effort, but if we've learned anything from reviewing studies, speaking with health professionals, and conducting years of our own trial and error, it's that you don't have to work out like a machine every day, sleep eight hours every night, or give up certain foods to feel good. Unless you're allergic to mangos. If you're allergic to mangos, you should probably not eat those. All you need is a solid understanding of what "healthy" looks like and strategies for navigating your current environment so that you can put some good habits in place. Habits that make sense for *you*. Habits that you can realistically stick to *most* of the time.

The first key to taking care of yourself in college? You have to want to. Your "give a shit" meter is the only thing that will *ever* dictate your ability to make positive changes in your life. Do you want to know how to avoid becoming pizza's bitch? How to consume alcohol so that you don't pass out and get wieners drawn on your face? How to exercise without dreading it? How to keep your cool when assignments start to pile up? How to get enough sleep so that your brain doesn't eat itself? If you're ready, then it's time to learn "how to not get fat in college" and so much more. **Let's do this.**

# CHAPTER 2

# FOOD

## JILL

**I used to moonlight as the mascot now and again back in high school.** Nothing builds character quite like a few hot hours in a giant pirate head coated with decades' worth of sweat. When I got to college, I wanted to utilize the invaluable entertainment skills I'd developed during my time as a gigantic human puppet. There seemed to be only one choice—I became a tour guide.

My tours were filled with bad jokes and awkward pauses. The only comment that consistently earned something other than pity laughter always happened in front of the dining hall, where I would talk about how fat I'd gotten since coming to college. While standing on a bench outside the entryway, I'd slap my belly for effect. "There's an all-you-can-eat buffet set up inside," I said, like a carnival worker trying to lure unsuspecting guests into the House of Horrors. "The food here is so good that I gained the Freshman 20!" Then I'd go on about how I had used all of my savings to buy new pants because I'd split the seams in the old ones. Apparently, the weight gain happened to everyone, so I wasn't embarrassed. And hey, at least I wasn't wearing a giant pirate head.

Google "Freshman 15," and you'll get nearly eighty million results. Many articles give seemingly simple yet unrealistic advice on how to avoid it: always walk to class, take the stairs instead of the elevator, don't eat a whole stick of butter. *Blah, blah, blah.* Others state it's entirely a myth—arguing that college weight gain is very minimal and actually the result of the physical transformation from a teen to an adult body. A second puberty of sorts? *Who knew?* There is some truth to that claim, because it is entirely normal and healthy to gain around five pounds during college as your body continues to change. For many, however, it's more than that. We spoke to a lot of students, and no one tried to blame their bodily changes on blossoming into an adult. Whether their weight gain was two pounds or fifteen, students were more than capable of zeroing in on how they were sabotaging their health. Some cited a total lack of exercise, others hard boozing, but an overwhelming majority declared that their rapidly expanding figure was a direct result of eating like a pig on Christmas. All of the food. All of the time. *All of it!*

> *"When I went in for my annual physical, I realized the Freshman 15 was real. Or the Freshman 22, in my case. I should have expected it, as I had been getting a tad bigger in the muffin top area."*
> —SAINT MARY'S COLLEGE OF CALIFORNIA, SOPHOMORE

In this chapter, we're going to give you a straightforward food rundown that will be less preachy than a typical health book and less dense and technical than a nutrition class. Dave and I still eat like shit sometimes, and we're going to argue that you should too. There are, however, some things that you should keep in mind when you're shoving things in your mouth, particularly given the excessive nature of the college environment. A categorization of foods based on their quality will be combined with some pointers on how to chow down, given the unfathomable amount of options you'll be exposed to. We'll also discuss strategies for experiencing *all of the food* in a way that won't make you feel like shit *all of the time.* Feasting at a buffet requires an awareness of portion control, so if you're hoping to hold onto your sweet precollege physique, stick around for that. And finally, we'll talk about cooking for yourself and the complications that can arise when food freedom becomes a reality.

## How to Choose When Faced with Choice

The typical dining situation in college is ridiculous. Much of your eating will happen at a buffet, which features endless options, lets you serve yourself, and doesn't give you a bill at the end. The food choices will span the entire nutritional spectrum, and if you've got

*"If I'm running late and don't have time to put together a good meal, sometimes I just grab one of the giant cookies by the register and eat that for dinner."*
—SARAH LAWRENCE COLLEGE, FRESHMAN

an unlimited item plan, you'll have the luxury of "sampling" whatever you want. A small handful of fries. A baby cup of soft serve. One teeny weeny slice of pizza on the side. Even on a pay-per-item plan, you may be tempted to opt for junk food because it's quick, cheap, and easy to eat.

To further complicate things, junk food is also absolutely delicious and is actually engineered to blow our minds. Most junk is high in salt, fat, and sugar. When any *one* of those ingredients is consumed independently, a pleasure response is triggered in our brains. Combine them, and your head explodes with delight. Research has shown that the brain's reward center essentially malfunctions when we eat foods high in fat and carbohydrates.[1] We crave those foods even when we're not hungry, and as one study suggests, human bodies haven't really evolved to handle that. That's probably why I can look at an apple after dinner and be like, "meh, don't need it," but moments later eye a box of Girl Scout Cookies and eat an entire sleeve. It's no wonder that 90 percent of adults don't eat enough real food[2]—junk food is the perfect drug. It's cheap, it's everywhere, it's delicious, it's addicting, *and* it's legal.

Assuming you're not regularly crushing Thin Mints by the dozen and brushing your teeth with Cool Whip, you probably don't need to avoid junk completely. If you don't have a serious health problem and can somewhat moderate your portions, crappy food isn't going to destroy your body. I ate a donut fifteen minutes before I sat down to write this. I know it's not good for me, but I was really feeling it, all smothered in pink frosting and topped with sprinkles. It looked incredible, and it needed a friend. A friend that was going to tear it apart and make it disappear. I was up to the task.

Donuts, however, don't make a regular appearance in my day or even my week. When I have a craving—when I see a donut that *must* be removed from this earth—I get after it, but I tend to avoid eating things that will make me physically feel like hot garbage twenty minutes later like that neon pink donut always will. I'm talking bloated and grumpy, with indigestion, heartburn, and maybe even some constipation thrown in for good measure. The "everything in moderation" adage might be overused, but it works when it comes to shitty food.

*"I don't think healthy eating means salad all the time, because if mac and cheese and chocolate cake are what I need emotionally to finish a 20-page paper, then I'm going to eat mac and cheese and cake. But eating that way every day for every meal eventually makes me sluggish and sad, and I'm pretty sure that is when it becomes unhealthy. I try to eat in a way that makes me feel good and gives me energy. I've realized that it's all about balance and listening to what my body wants and needs."*
—GEORGETOWN UNIVERSITY, FRESHMAN

But let's face it: self-control is challenging to master. I don't see donuts every day, which is part of the reason I don't eat them more often. The college environment, however, ups the ante. It's easy to go buck wild when you are always surrounded by temptation.

The good news: You don't have to eat *anything* in moderation if you don't want to. There will be no one to prevent you from eating a whole bucket of fries at lunch every day if that's what you dream about. You are now entirely responsible for making your own choices when it comes to food.

The bad news: You are now entirely responsible for making your own choices when it comes to food! No matter how much you might want to, you should *not* eat a whole bucket of fries every day at lunch, you filthy monster! Those salty pleasure sticks may be unassuming at first, but eating copious amounts of fries, or whatever else you crave, every day will ultimately become a hard-to-break ritual. Unfortunately, it's all on *you* to make sure that doesn't happen, because no one will be there to smack those bad boys out of your greasy hands.

Like it or not, balance is crucial if you want to be healthy. You should have fun with what you eat, but you also don't want to treat every day like a free-for-all. A basic understanding of food and some simple guidelines for how to eat well will get you one step closer to locking that shit down.

## This Is Not a Diet

Before we dive in, I have to clarify something. Our primary objective with this chapter is to encourage you to eat well for health, not for weight loss. It's easy to think that those two go hand in hand, but that's not always the case. The one you emphasize *really* matters. Prioritizing weight loss doesn't guarantee you'll be eating properly. Many diets focus on restrictions—don't eat this, don't eat that—which can make eating *anywhere* stressful. More importantly, it's not sustainable for the long haul

*"As a freshman, it is your first taste of freedom in all aspects, but especially in nutrition. You find yourself being able to eat whatever you want, from burgers every meal to cereal for dinner."*
—UNIVERSITY OF SOUTHERN CALIFORNIA, SOPHOMORE

and doesn't result in lasting change. Research shows that the lost weight comes back for most dieters, within as little as a few months.[3] In essence, cutting out everything "bad" and eating exclusively what's "good" isn't effective. It might seem doable for a few months, but it's not a realistic template for life. So why even bother starting there? Drop any plans that focus on what you *shouldn't* eat. Healthy eating doesn't mean eating healthy food all the time. It means that you approach food with a degree of flexibility and listen to your body for feedback as to how you're doing, not the scale or some food dogma. So instead of trapping yourself inside some temporary diet that won't help you in the long run, make a concerted effort to develop a healthy relationship with food. Getting there isn't always quick, but once you figure it out, that relationship will serve you for the rest of your life. The best part? Your weight will absolutely stay in check as a result.

Now, I say all of this knowing full well that flexible eating can be daunting at first—it certainly took me some time to figure out. I started CrossFit shortly after college, right around the time Paleo was becoming popular and bacon was being hailed as the king of all proteins. The pigs were terrified. Anyway, I initially really liked the black-and-white approach of Paleo, which was to give up all grains, sugar, and dairy. I was convinced that I'd get a sweet six-pack if I jumped on the bandwagon. So, I went for it. Did I get that six-pack? No. Instead, I developed gigantic man quads from all the protein and powerlifting, alongside a real obsession with bacon. I had to buy new pants . . . again. *Curses!*

Given that wasn't really the look I had set out to achieve, I decided against a dietary life that forbid bread, ice cream, and cheese. I really love those foods, and having to ignore their existence at every turn was a bummer. I moved away from a restrictive version of Paleo after about six months, though ultimately, I had learned a valuable lesson: my body *felt* different. I actually felt great. I experienced heightened energy levels when I cut back on sugar and introduced more vegetables and protein to my diet. I had given my body something different, and it had communicated approval. The whole Paleo experiment didn't help me get washboard abs, but it did give me a more definite sense of *what* to eat and *how* to make changes. Since bailing on Paleo, I've stayed entirely away from food restrictions; however, I eat certain foods—the ones that zap my energy—less frequently than I used to. I have a clearer sense of which foods make my body feel great and now intentionally plan my meals around those. Ultimately, I now crave the way I feel after eating quality foods, and that alone prevents me from constantly stuffing my face with shitty ones.

My point is twofold. Don't diet or restrict, but do experiment with different ways of eating. Give your body two or three weeks to respond with feedback after you make changes. As we said earlier, the key is learning to recognize the warning signs. Puffy, sweaty, tired, sad, or shitting mud? If this is you after eating, it's time for a change. Energized and upbeat? That means you've properly fueled for battle (or class). Your body will tell you which foods it thrives on and which it merely tolerates—all you have to do is pay attention and adjust accordingly. With some guidance for your trial-and-error process, we hope that you will discover a balanced and healthy way to eat that will make you feel good.

## What to Eat

The following list is a starting point for your experimenting and has been assembled with the help of a registered dietitian. The groupings are meant to clarify which foods pack the most nutritional punch. No one food is going to kill you or torpedo your health goals, but certain foods are best as daily staples, whereas others are better

# WHAT TO EAT

| | |
|---|---|
| **EVERYDAY** | All fruits, all veggies, most proteins (chicken, seafood, pork, beef, eggs, turkey, tofu, tempeh), whole grains (rice, quinoa, unflavored oatmeal), beans, all nuts and natural nut butters, avocado, olives, quality fats (olive oil, coconut oil, butter), plain yogurt, plain kefir, cottage cheese, bread products without preservatives, real cheese, milk |
| | *These are real foods. Most are grown or raised and can be found in nature. They will rot if you forget them in the back of your mini fridge. Many are colorful. These are the most nutrient-dense foods you can consume.* |
| **SOMETIMES** | Pizza, bacon, flavored oatmeal, packaged bread/bagels, tortillas, pasta, cereal/granola, cream, sour cream, industrial vegetable & seed oils, processed peanut butter, microwave popcorn, bottled smoothies, homemade sweets |
| | *Many of these foods contain high levels of saturated fat or sugar. Some are factory made. Although these foods are less than perfect, they still offer some nutritional value.* |
| **RARELY** | Chips, fries, fruit juice, ice cream, processed meats and cheeses, soda, sugary teas, candy bars, packaged sweets (like muffins, cookies, cakes), fast food |
| | *These aren't foods, these are products. They are loaded with chemicals and/or sugar. These offer the least nutrients or no nutrients at all.* |

as occasional additions. I'm guessing it's obvious from the naming conventions, but you'll be doing your body a solid if you routinely eat the "everyday" foods, as these are the ones that will give you the most energy. Then, mix in items from the "sometimes" and "rarely" categories as desired throughout the week. These might not add to your energy stores, but they'll make you happy inside, and that's just as important.

It's hopefully clear by now that you will likely have unlimited access to the foods listed above. Particularly the foods in the last two sections. And that access complicates matters. No one is losing their minds over the all-you-can-eat broccoli, but it's definitely hard to eat pizza only *sometimes* when you walk by it *every day*. If your diet consists mostly of foods found in the "sometimes" or "rarely" categories, start making some simple swaps. Even if you feel fine surviving off of fries and pizza and avoiding vegetables, you're not giving your body what it needs to function properly. It's as simple as that. This shit is *science*! Food is a central component of our well-being, and if you're not getting the right stuff, you'll have no idea how good your body can really feel. If you eat better, you'll be able to climb up walls, shoot webs from your wrists, and Tarzan your way through the city from building to building. Or something similar. Anyway, make some changes, but keep in mind that they don't need to be to the tune of a complete and speedy overhaul. Start small by adding in or making a daily trade for food in the "everyday" category. The following strategies will guide that process.

## How to Eat

These guidelines aren't revolutionary; you've likely heard some of them before. They work, though, which is why they've stuck around. Treat them like you would any other rule, letting them guide your decision making when you're trying to eat well, and throwing them out the window every so often to keep your sanity. Here are eight to keep in mind:

1.  **Eat Your Colors.** Take your current fruit and vegetable consumption and double it. More than half of college students only eat one or two total servings of fruits and vegetables per day,[4] well below the CDC daily recommendation of 1½–2 cups of fruits and 2–3 cups of vegetables, which equates to between 5 and 8 servings of both. As nutritional powerhouses, they should be the foundation of your diet. Fruits and veggies are jam-packed with vitamins and minerals that boost immunity and protect against chronic disease. The goodness found inside kale and spinach keeps your bones strong and your teeth from crumbling. Bananas, broccoli, and cucumbers carry potassium, which helps your muscles rebuild, and carrots, bell peppers, sweet potatoes, and tomatoes are vessels for vitamin A, which is what powers your peepers. All

    *"Sometimes you've just gotta eat those undercooked greens."*
    —UNIVERSITY OF ROCHESTER, FRESHMAN

    veggies and fruits are carbohydrates, which provide you with the energy you need to breathe, walk, type, eat, think, dance the robot, or hold thirty pounds of textbooks . . . just a few of the things you need to do to survive college. Fill half of your plate with colored food first, then fill the other half with a split of whole grains and protein. If cooked veggies aren't your thing, opt for raw ones from the salad bar instead.

If the produce choices at your school aren't of good quality, speak up. Talk to the head of your dining hall. I'm serious! Don't write a crappy review bashing your school's food on some third-party website. Instead, reach out via email and then schedule a meeting. Be respectful and give useful feedback—it's the most effective way to get what you need. It's also in the best interest of the institution to make sure that its students feel heard and are satisfied with what's offered, which is precisely why they will make changes when possible. Advocating for yourself is an essential life skill, particularly regarding things that impact the quality of your daily life.

2. **Eat at Mealtimes.** "Fourthmeal" was an ad campaign used by a particular fast-food taco chain back in the mid-2000s to attract hordes of stoners and drunk

# MACRONUTRIENTS

Each macronutrient plays an important role in the functioning of your body. While it's not necessary that you "count" macros, it's important that you include each type in your diet regularly.

| | CARBS | PROTEINS | FATS |
|---|---|---|---|
| **PRIMARY FUNCTIONS** | Supply cells with energy<br>*the brain and red blood cells can only be powered by glucose*<br><br>Can be stored as energy for later use<br><br>Help preserve muscle<br>*when your body is low on the necessary glucose, your muscles may be broken down to provide emergency energy* | Builds bones, muscles, cartilage, skin, hair, and nails<br><br>Repairs tissue after exercise or injury<br><br>Regulates hormones<br><br>Helps with digestion and curbs hunger | Secondary source of energy<br>*significantly more oxygen is required to break down fat than carbs*<br><br>Regulates body temperature<br><br>Important for vitamin absorption and storage<br>*Vitamins A, D, E, and K cannot function without fat* |
| **SELECT FOODS** | *Fruit, Veggies, Grains* | *Meats* | *Oils, Avocado* |
| | | *Nuts & Nut Butters, Quality Full-Fat Dairy Products, Eggs* | |
| | *Beans, Chickpeas, Quinoa, Lentils* | | |
| | *most junk foods live in the intersection between carbs and fats* | | |

people to stop in for late-night chalupas. It promoted a full dinner's worth of dinner . . . after dinner. Even though there's nothing better than eating the shit out of a chalupa at midnight on occasion, daily or weekly indulgence in second dinner *isn't* one of the secrets of highly successful people. If you're regularly hungry late at night, that means you're not eating enough during the day. To start, eat breakfast, even if it's small. Then eat a substantial lunch, snack between meals, and have dinner at dinnertime. If you tend to be rushed in the evening and hungry at night because your dining hall closes early, keep some smuggled fruit in your room so that you're prepared when hunger strikes.

3. **Snack Well.** I've always hated the word "snack." I can't say it without aggressively wrinkling my nose, and seeing it in print gives me the creeps. Snacks, however, are genius—they're basically tiny insurance policies that prevent us from going nuts at our next meal. They allow for sustained energy throughout the day, which can be a lifesaver when you're bouncing between class, homework, and a job. Combine a quality carbohydrate and a protein or fat to ensure maximum satiation, and try to only eat snacks when you're actually hungry, not just bored.

## PERFECT SNACK COMBOS

| EASY-TO-EAT CARBOHYDRATE | PROTEIN OR FAT SIDEKICK |
|---|---|
| Carrot or celery sticks | Peanut/almond butter |
| Cucumber slices | Plain yogurt |
| Bell pepper strips | Hummus |
| Pretzels | Cheese stick |
| Berries | Almonds |
| Apple | Jerky |
| Banana | Hard-boiled egg |
| Clementines | Olives |

4. **Eat Your Calories, Don't Drink Them.** Liquid calories don't fill you up like solid ones, and most drinks are devoid of any nutritional benefit and full of sugar. Cut back on soda, chocolate milk, sweet tea, juice, and fancy coffee drinks. If you're reading this while sipping on a hot, creamy, delicious mocha, (a) thank you for reading, but (b) stop drinking that sugary death bomb! Well, not really, but at least don't have it every day. Not only does it likely have more sugar than ice cream, it's also expensive. Opt for a black coffee instead, and splash in some milk if you need it. Try sticking to water, sparkling water, coffee, and unsweetened tea (hot or iced) for a few weeks. You'll notice the difference in your stomach and your wallet.

5. **Eat Real Food.** There's only a one-letter discrepancy between produce and product, but there's a world of difference. Food is an industry, and unfortunately, the goal of food manufacturers isn't to ensure your good health, it's to make money. Companies spend millions of dollars each year trying to convince consumers that a product is healthy, *especially* when it's not. Because it's remarkably easy to be fooled, your best defense is a bit of awareness.

   "Health food" marketing ploys began in the early seventies when scientific studies first connected a healthy diet to the prevention of cancer and other diseases. Companies saw a business opportunity and took it, putting bold and typically unwarranted claims about the healthfulness of their products on the packaging. The nutrition label, in part, was created as a way to regulate that type of marketing,[5] but many companies still use deceptive packaging to draw people in, assuming that we won't read the label if we believe a product is healthy.

   Protect yourself by ignoring any wellness claims or "greenwashed" packaging that makes you *assume* something is good for you, and approach foods that are actively advertised to you with caution. Regardless of how kind or honest they may seem, commercials are designed to get you to spend money, not to make informed decisions. Get into the habit of reading the ingredient list on the back of the package and follow two basic rules. First, the shorter the list, the better (typically). Second, if you can't pronounce or visualize an ingredient, chances are good that it was created in a lab, so best to skip that product.

*Three Red Flags. Keep an eye out for these particular ingredients in your food. They're the worst of the worst.*

- **Butylated hydroxyanisole (BHA)** is a preservative often found in breakfast cereal, nut mixes, chewing gum, butter spread, meat, dehydrated potatoes, dessert and beverage mixes, popcorn, chips, and beer. It's also used to create animal feed, food packaging, makeup, and rubber and petroleum products. A real multipurpose ingredient, am I right?! BHA is *not* banned in the US but is banned in Japan and many European countries, including the UK. Even though California includes BHA on a list of "Known Carcinogens and Reproductive Toxicants" (also known as the Prop 65 list) due to its link to cancer,[6] it still somehow passes muster with the FDA. Terrifying.
- **Potassium bromate** is an additive found in many packaged bread products. It has been linked to kidney and nervous system damage, thyroid and GI tract issues, and cancer.[7] Potassium bromate is *not* banned in the US but is banned in all of Europe, Canada, and China. Just like BHA, it was added to the Prop 65 list in 1990 due to cancer links.
- **Artificial colors** are apparent in certain foods. Bright drinks, candies, and some cereals clearly have an added tint, but so can salmon, yogurt, salad dressing, pickles, popcorn, granola and protein bars, soups, and canned fruit. Eight dyes—including Red 40, Blue 2, and Yellow 5 (all of which can go by complicated aliases)—have been linked to cancer and hyperactivity in children.[8] Artificial colors are *not* banned in the US but are banned in Norway, Finland, France, Austria, and the UK.

6. **Cut Back on Added Sugar.** Any idea how much sugar the average American consumes each day? For the purpose of your guessing, let me tell you that the recommended daily sugar allowance is thirty-six grams for men and twenty-four grams for women. You ready to guess? All right. Here's the answer: seventy grams.[9] That's a half cup of sugar. Every. Single. Day. *Holy shit.* That's

not just disgusting, it's also scary because an abundance of fructose can actually damage the liver just like too much alcohol can. In the last fifty years, world-wide sugar consumption has tripled.[10]

Unfortunately, there's no real end in sight. Sugar isn't regulated in the same way that other toxic substances, like booze and tobacco, are. Quite the contrary. It's practically been built into our food system. Added sugar is in 75 percent of packaged items.[11] You'll find between twenty and forty grams in desserts and sodas, which shouldn't be a surprise, but what might shock you is that you'll find nearly the same amount in muffins, flavored yogurt, cereals, and granola bars. The only way to know for sure what you're getting yourself into is to read the nutrition label on whatever you're eating. While you're there, check out the ingredient list. Items are displayed in order of predominance, and it will blow your mind how often you'll find sugar in the top three.

Thinking sugar-free is the way to go? Think again. Although five artificial sweeteners are considered safe by the FDA, research suggests that the daily consumption of diet sodas—one of the most popular vessels of fake sugar—actually *increases* the risk of metabolic syndrome and diabetes by 36 and 67 percent, respectively.[12] Those are the exact diseases we should be trying to avoid by cutting back on real sugar, so it appears the fake stuff isn't really helping us out in regard to our health.

Fruit, however, doesn't register in the same way as sugar. The twenty grams of sweetness in an apple, for instance, don't count toward the daily limit stated earlier. That's because apples, and all other fruits, are perfectly packaged with fiber, vitamins, and minerals that positively alter the way your body processes glucose. You should eat fruit without concern, so long as it's whole and not juiced or dried. Avoid bottled smoothies that advertise themselves as having two apples, half a banana, and a quarter cup of blue-berries. While the label will shout "no added sugar," there's also no fiber to slow down the digestion of glucose. That was stripped from the fruit when it was obliterated and jammed into a bottle. Therefore, your body processes all fifty-three grams of that fruit sugar no differently than it would process the sugar in a milkshake.

Some argue that sugar is the most toxic ingredient in our food today.[14] Both the real and fake versions offer zero nutritional benefits, and overeating them can lead to a whole host of terrifying medical conditions. Furthermore, it's incredibly addictive (some studies say *as* addictive as cocaine), so it's a hard habit to break if you get sucked in.[15] The bottom line is that we *all* need to be mindful of our sugar consumption. If sugar has become a regular part of your day, especially unintentionally, now is a good time to start eliminating some of it wherever you can. Conscious consumption is key.

---

**Sweet Nicknames.** You may not be able to locate "sugar" easily, as it's often listed under an alias. Here are the sixty-one different names that it can go by:

"Agave nectar, Barbados sugar, Barley malt, Barley malt syrup, Beet sugar, Brown sugar, Buttered syrup, Cane juice, Cane juice crystals, Cane sugar, Caramel, Carob syrup, Castor sugar, Coconut palm sugar, Coconut sugar, Confectioners' sugar, Corn sweetener, Corn syrup, Corn syrup solids, Date sugar, Dehydrated cane juice, Demerara sugar, Dextrin, Dextrose, Evaporated cane juice, Free-flowing brown sugars, Fructose, Fruit juice, Fruit juice concentrate, Glucose, Glucose solids, Golden sugar, Golden syrup, Grape sugar, HFCS (High-Fructose Corn Syrup), Honey, Icing sugar, Invert sugar, Malt syrup, Maltodextrin, Maltol, Maltose, Mannose, Maple syrup, Molasses, Muscovado, Organic Sugar, Palm sugar, Panocha, Powdered sugar, Raw sugar, Refiner's syrup, Rice syrup, Saccharose, Sorghum Syrup, Sucrose, Sugar (granulated), Sweet Sorghum, Syrup, Treacle, Turbinado sugar, Yellow sugar."[13]

7.  **Don't Start Sweet.** Speaking of sugar, there's really no better way to guarantee a midday struggle than to start with sweets for breakfast. Sugar-heavy breakfasts—think pancakes, muffins, scones, waffles, cereal, bagels, toast with jam, sweetened yogurt, granola—cause a quick spike in your blood sugar. Your body loves this, as your blood sugar is low in the morning, and sugar provides an energy boost. Unfortunately, within a couple of hours, you'll likely experience a crash, indicated by fatigue, irritability, headache, and difficulty concentrating. You'll feel terrible until you get *more* sugar. To avoid that never-ending shitstorm, get a good dose of protein and fat at breakfast instead with things like eggs, avocado, nut butter, and Greek yogurt.

## SUGAR CONTENT IN COMMON FOODS

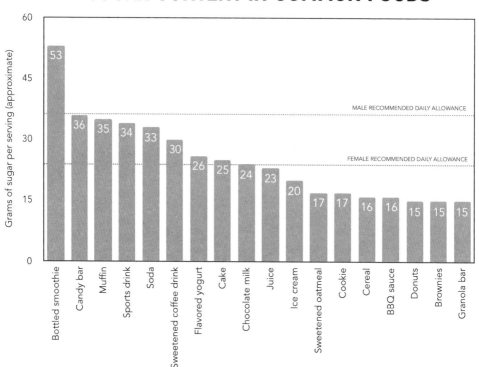

8. **Eat at a B+.** You won't be able to avoid unhealthy choices all the time, nor should you. The world is filled with delicious and terrible foods that should be enjoyed by those who want them. Kicking off the morning with a bacon, egg, and cheese on a bagel or capping off the night with an enormous bowl of ice cream sometimes just feels like the right move. So, I sometimes do it and then adjust accordingly. If I already ate or know I am going to eat some mouthwatering garbage-food, I will intentionally eat well for the rest of the day. I've found that if I freely allow myself to give in to temptation, I'm less likely to go overboard because I know I'll be able to eat that food again the next time I'm craving it. Balancing those choices with healthier foods is how I regularly hit a "B+" with my nutrition, which keeps me feeling healthy, unrestricted, and free from guilt. The closest comparison is probably budgeting. On a limited amount of money, you can't buy everything you want all at once. So you learn to spread out big purchases and try to spend thoughtfully and intentionally in between. Food can be looked at the same way—permit yourself to indulge once a day or a few times a week without any guilt by consciously making quality choices the rest of the time. Food can provide *both* the needed fuel and desired pleasure if you focus on balancing spontaneity with discipline.

## Indulge Like a Pro

Eating with reckless abandon is part of the college experience for many. I remember the first time I ate an entire family-sized bag of Cheetos by myself. I made it three-quarters of the way through before I even thought to assess my pillaging. When I realized how few neon-orange puffs remained, I was actually impressed with myself. I sat in that moment for a second and then proceeded to polish off the entire thing. *Just a regular Tuesday.*

> *"When I first got to college, I saw all of this food, just staring me in the face. I had soft serve every night."*
>
> —TUFTS UNIVERSITY, FRESHMAN

Restraint wasn't on my radar when I got to college, but even if it had been, it's challenging to exhibit self-control when surrounded by unlimited quantities of all the foods you crave. Unless your family is in the ice cream business, navigating constant temptation is probably a new experience, and setting some ground rules can keep you from becoming a complete animal. Here are seven ways to do that:

1. **Reserve Treats for Special Occasions.** Food provides comfort. It gives us a way to let loose, socialize, have fun, celebrate, and commiserate, all without substantial effort. Hard day? Have a burrito. Great day? Have some cake. Rewarding yourself with certain foods on special occasions is a common practice.

   This policy becomes problematic, however, when every day is viewed as a celebration. Back away from the food holiday calendar, where January first is National Bloody Mary Day, the second is National Cream Puff Day, the third is National Chocolate-Covered Cherry Day, the fourth is National Spaghetti Day, and the fifth is National Whipped Cream Day. *This is just January.* What a way to start the year! Bet you're not thinking about resolutions on day five while you're squirting whipped cream into your mouth straight from the can.

   Allow celebrations to feel special by not celebrating every day—at least not with food. Given that breakfast and lunch are unlikely celebratory meals, eat well at those times from Monday through Friday to give yourself more leeway at dinner and over the weekend.

2. **Don't Deprive Yourself.** Years ago, during one of our many *attempts* to get shredded, Dave and I tested out a weekly "cheat day." We'd eat *perfectly* from Sunday morning through Friday night, and then as soon as our workout was over on Saturday morning, we'd lose our minds. After all, we'd spent an entire week thinking about the foods we'd been missing. There was pressure to make every moment count when cheat day finally arrived, so we did just that. *9:00 a.m.— breakfast burritos, iced mochas, and cookies. 1:00 p.m.—foot-long Italian subs and chips. 6:00 p.m.—lots of pizza and lots of beer. 9:00 p.m.—ice cream sundaes; more cookies.*

   Sunday morning was always a real kick in the face. Our bodies were on overdrive, trying to sort out the cesspool we'd created in our stomachs during the previous twenty-four hours. We not only ate an obscene amount of trash, but we also didn't include a single healthy item (a waste of precious stomach space!). I look at this now and think, *Man, we were idiots*, but it took us *months* to figure out that what we were doing was unhealthy. The cheat day system doesn't work for many because it removes "the rules" after a long stretch of restriction—a recipe for disaster if you have trouble with self-control.

3.  **Don't Indulge in the Same Thing More Than Two Days in a Row.** A treat, by definition, is an item that is out of the ordinary and gives great pleasure. So let your treats be treats. Don't let ice cream become your automatic postdinner routine. By spacing out your indulgences, you give yourself a chance to look forward to them, which in turn allows each one to feel special.

4.  **Avoid Desperation.** Keep healthy food in your backpack or room to prevent a situation where you're starving and, as a result, grab the first thing you can get your hands on—which, when you're desperate, will likely be something packaged, comforting, and terrible for you. Indulgences are much more enjoyable when they happen due to choice rather than desperation.

5.  **Plan for When You're Drunk.** As you'll learn in the alcohol chapter, drunk munching doesn't help sober you up, which was absolutely a misconception of mine during freshman year. I once ate a whole loaf of white bread in my top bunk after a night of hard drinking, thinking it would stop the world from spinning around me. It didn't. I puked up a stomach of coconut rum and sandwich slices in my roommate's tiny trash can, then passed out covered in crumbs.

Eating after a night out can be part of the fun, but if impaired judgment results in your choices or portions being out of control, then attack your weakness head-on by devising a system to help you avoid overdoing it. Keep popcorn, pretzels, instant noodles, or a decently healthy cereal in your dorm room, so you've got something to eat when you get home. If you're going out, split a meal with a friend and order a comfort food that has a dash of something good, like a thin-crust veggie pizza or a grilled chicken sandwich. Those calories aren't serving any purpose in terms of alcohol

> "I've stopped bringing money with me when I go out, and I don't keep food in my room so that I don't eat after I've been drinking."
> —COLLEGE OF WILLIAM & MARY, JUNIOR

defense, so try to consume something that won't add to how shitty you're going to feel when you wake up.

6.  **Steer Clear of Temptations.** If you don't want to eat dessert and fries every day, don't curiously saunter past those stations in the dining hall. If you don't want to eat chips at night, don't keep an emergency stockpile in your dorm room. A study published in 2012 about self-control in the face of desire stated that situational factors, more than personality, affect someone's ability to refrain from temptation.[16] In short, we humans are weak-willed and programmed to fail. *Which is exactly why the robots will win.* The difference between those who cave and those who don't? **Access.** When bad options abound, you're much more likely to crave them. So, maintain some distance between yourself and the "rarely" or "occasional" foods that you typically have trouble resisting.

*"When I was living at home, there was rarely unhealthy food in the house, which made it a lot easier to eat well. In college, you always have the option of ice cream after dinner, or even ice cream for dinner if you want. Having the option requires more self-control, and that is a hard transition to make."*
—WASHINGTON UNIVERSITY, FRESHMAN

7.  **Don't Throw in the Towel.** So you cracked. You ate a whole pizza at 2:00 a.m. Don't let a single indiscretion snowball into an avalanche of not-great-for-your-health decisions. Continuing to indulge because you feel like you've already ruined your day is like continuing to spend money that you don't have by putting your purchases on a credit card. It all adds up. But here's the thing—you *will* overdo it at some point. You and pizza are going to have a standoff, and pizza will win. Pizza is a powerful opponent, and you should not judge yourself for losing the battle. Remember, it was just one battle—not the whole war. Start fresh tomorrow. Work out, drink lots of water, eat a healthy breakfast, and stop feeling guilty! The best thing that you can do now is to take note of whatever you're feeling and stash it away. You're going to get another opportunity to battle, and now you're one step closer to avoiding becoming pizza's bitch . . . again.

**Detox with Water.** Your kidneys are responsible for dealing with the mess that exists in your body when you've gone a little wild with unhealthy foods. Kidneys filter blood, a job that requires them to essentially snatch up anything nasty and send it out with pee. But kidneys can't do their crucial job without water, and they do it best when water is available in excess.[17] Keep this in mind when you go off the deep end with any foods that you know don't sit well in your body, and instead of feeling shitty about yourself, counter your actions by drinking a huge bottle of water. Dilution fights pollution.

## Quantity Control

A 2016 study found that 75 percent of Americans classified their diet as good, great, or excellent,[18] yet 70 percent of our country is overweight, and more than half of that group is considered obese.[19] Where's the disconnect? Many registered dietitians believe that people are either (a) falling for "health" food marketing on unhealthy foods or (b) not observing proper portion sizes.

Coming face-to-face with a buffet three times a day when you're on your own for the first time can make food feel even more overwhelming. Not only do you have to make choices about what to put on your plate, you also have to consider how much. Without considering portion size, it's remarkably easy to overeat despite your best intentions. One of my friends recently started tracking her food for a health challenge and realized that she was consuming a thousand more calories each day than she thought, simply because her portions were too large.

I've never been a dainty eater. When I was in sixth grade, my summer camp counselor sent a letter home to my parents that read: "Jill needs to learn to control herself when it's time for seconds in the dining hall." It's possible that comment was in response to a minor incident where I *accidentally* hockey checked a kid who was picking up the very last chicken patty. He dropped it, and I ate it off the floor.

*"When I first started college, I found it hard to limit my intake as I wanted to try everything and maximize each swipe used to get into the dining hall."*
—UNIVERSITY OF CALIFORNIA, LOS ANGELES, FRESHMAN

Being healthy in college was a challenge not just because I always wanted seconds, but because I wanted to sample *everything*. Suddenly I was surrounded by an array of delicious options, all of which I had never experienced unfettered access to before. I found it hard not to load up my plate every time I was in the dining hall. I only got better with restraint when I figured out how to listen to my body, which took a ridiculously long time. *Welp, I feel like trash again. Probably didn't need that fifth slice of pizza.* You don't have to suffer through stomachache after stomachache to get a handle on portion control, though. Here are four ways to consider serving size that don't require a physical sacrifice:

1. **Estimate Portion Size.** Ever participated in the classic "how many jellybeans are in this humongous glass jar" game? Anyone who is out to win probably devises a system, like say, ballpark the number of jellybeans on the bottom layer, estimate the number of layers in the jar, crank out a quick little multiplication, and boom: a guess that's sure to win. *I've never won.* Even if you've never played that classic raffle game, you're probably no stranger to approximate measurement. For a guess to be "educated," a system is critical. Eyeballing *is* an efficient and decently accurate system, so long as you have something concrete to use for comparison.[20]

   Your hands work particularly well as a frame of reference when it comes to food, because, unless you've got hooks for hands, they're always with you. *I'm sorry if you have hand hooks, I bet that's really hard.* Your feet work if you're measuring the size of a room but are better left under the table when it comes to eating. Furthermore, if any of your portions are even close to the size of your feet, you'd better be in some sort of competition. *For your first challenge, a boot of mashed potatoes!*

   The size of your palm, your thumb, your fist, and so forth will obviously be different than someone else's, but that difference is actually okay, as it should equate to the amount that is appropriate for your needs. A five-two woman should have a smaller hand than a six-two man, thus her portions will be smaller than his, which they probably should be. He burns more calories than she does each day by simply being alive, so he needs more food. Thus, this *handy* system (see what I did there) is a solid way of measuring food.

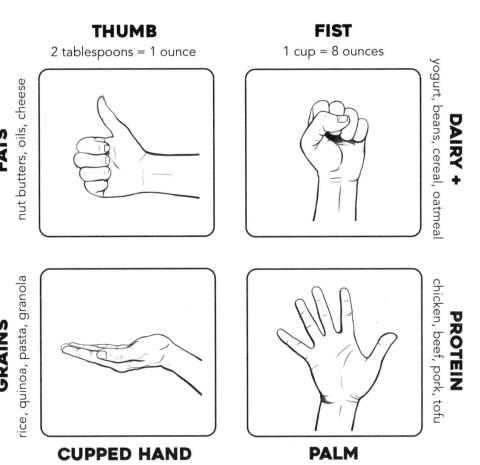

**THUMB**
2 tablespoons = 1 ounce

**FIST**
1 cup = 8 ounces

**FATS**
nut butters, oils, cheese

**DAIRY +**
yogurt, beans, cereal, oatmeal

**GRAINS**
rice, quinoa, pasta, granola

**PROTEIN**
chicken, beef, pork, tofu

**CUPPED HAND**
1/2 cup = 4 ounces

**PALM**
~1/3 cup = 3 ounces

2. **Push Some Water and Watch the Clock Before Pressing "Repeat."** The curse of the buffet is that you can finish one plate and jump right back up for another without a moment of hesitation. Maybe you ran up a mountain and need that second plate of food, but maybe you're just bored and want to see how many burgers you can eat in one sitting. Before hitting the buffet a second time, drink a full glass of water (hell, make it two!) and set a timer for five minutes before determining whether you're actually still hungry.

3. **Listen to Your Body.** Your body knows things. It is designed to tell you when you're consuming a food that it doesn't like, or when you've had too much food altogether. Ever felt bloated, gassy, hot, and uncomfortable at the end of the meal? Oh. No? Yeah . . . me neither. That's your body communicating that you've overeaten—you just need to be present enough to listen. If you need to unbutton your pants after eating, it's probably time to cut back on your portions. Not that I really know from experience. I swear. I only did that once. In an Olive Garden. I just went a little overboard on the free breadsticks and needed some room to move, all right!?

4. **Eat What You Need.** Unfortunately, it's easy for us to tune out our bodies because we're often preoccupied with socializing while we eat. Additionally, it's possible to be influenced by the group that you're eating with.

> *"Who I have meals with always impacts what and how much I eat. I eat way more than I need to when I'm with the baseball players, and eat much healthier food than usual when I'm with a girl that I'm into."*
> —PITZER COLLEGE, FRESHMAN

Make an effort to eat what you need. You're the one putting food into your mouth (hopefully), and you're the one that will be stuck feeling like trash if you overdo it. You're in charge of your consumption, for better or worse. Is it hard to eat a reasonable portion when everyone around you is housing plates of fries and stacks of chicken patties? It definitely can be, but try your best to do you. Resist the urge to do what everyone around you is doing with their food. Once you've got a success or two under your belt, you'll know it's possible and will be able to do it *again* with less stress. And then *again*. And *again*. Before you know it, what and how much the people around you are eating won't matter.

## Cooking for One

If you're lucky, you'll have access to a kitchen at some point during college. Not one of those nasty dorm situations with sticky counters, ancient hot plates, and spaghetti-splattered microwaves. I mean the real deal. An actual temple of cooking, complete with a stove top, an oven, and some proper tools.

The privilege of a kitchen presents both benefits and challenges. Being able to determine what goes into your meals is a major health perk, but spending time and money on cooking and food shopping when you would rather spend that time and money literally anywhere else can be a real bummer. The reality, however, is that unless you work at Google or an equally badass company that has a cafeteria to provide you with meals, dining halls will be a thing of the past once you graduate.

*"Word to the wise, not knowing how to cook is the biggest turnoff in the world. You're an adult, google it and get it done."*
—NEW YORK UNIVERSITY, RECENT GRAD

Beyond being able to advertise your culinary skills on dating apps, there's a lot to gain by learning how to make yourself food while in college. Although cooking at home requires time and planning, it's truly the best option for your health and wallet. The trick is figuring out how to make it quick, cheap, and fun.

## Keep it Quick

The first key to enjoying cooking is to make something that you're excited to eat. The second key is to get it into your belly as soon as possible. Don't place unrealistic expectations on yourself in terms of how much time you'll be able to dedicate to the creation of sustenance. If you want to avoid or cut back on fast food, focus on fast meals instead. Here are three ways to do that:

- **Don't Stray from Simple:** Plan to make dishes and recipes that don't require a lot of ingredients, as that means there will be less to prep, clean, and buy. Additionally, zero in on recipes that can be completed in under twenty minutes. It's easy to quit altogether with cooking if it becomes complicated, expensive, and time consuming. When you're busy and stressed, convenience has a sneaky way of trumping health. Take advantage of the tons of cookbooks and blogs that specialize in quick, cheap meals, and if you really love cooking, then turn labor-intensive meals into weekend activities and share the workload with friends.

- **Buy an Instant Pot:** There's nothing better than coming home to a meal that's already made. There are three ways to achieve this: (1) move back in with your parents, (2) find yourself an outstanding roommate, or (3) buy a slow cooker or Instant Pot. One is not ideal, two is hard to find, and three is fifty dollars. Once or twice a week, take five minutes to load up your robotic cooking device before class, and you'll come home to dinner and lunch for days, all with minimal hassle. Chicken breast and a sauce of your choice go in in the morning, shredded chicken to throw on anything comes out at night. The best thing about an Instant Pot in particular is that it's also a pressure cooker, so if you forgot to load it up before class, it can still be used to make a meal at night. Additionally, it can cook rice and steam veggies. I bet it could even wash your dirty socks, but that's really gross and may result in a house fire, so you probably should use the laundry room instead.

- **Have a Quick Signature Dish:** Identify a few meals you'll always be psyched to eat that are (a) reasonably healthy, (b) use ingredients you typically have on hand, and (c) can be prepared in under five minutes. This is critical for when you've had a busy day and won't have much time to cook or when you get home and need food immediately but haven't planned ahead. Think scrambled eggs and toast. A quesadilla and a handful of bagged salad. Greek yogurt, fruit, and granola. Frozen mac and cheese and some sliced cucumbers. You get the gist.

*"The only reason I ate vegetables at home was because my parents made me. Eating the same way at college has been a struggle. There are so many delicious (and unhealthy) options here."*

—CARLETON COLLEGE, SOPHOMORE

## Keep it Cheap

Obviously, preparing food in your own kitchen is more affordable than eating out, but that doesn't remove the simple fact that spending money on ingredients brings much less joy than ordering a pizza. Here are three ways to keep your grocery bill under control:

- **Plant-Heavy:** Fruits and many veggies can be snacked on raw, and those that can't normally cook up quickly, satisfying the "quick" requirement from before. On top of that, though, produce is a cheap centerpiece when compared to animal protein. Plan your meals around hearty vegetables such as zucchini, potatoes, eggplant, mushrooms, and broccoli, then add on other inexpensive plant-based ingredients like canned beans and whole grains. Look to eggs, tofu, Greek yogurt, canned tuna, and ground chicken, turkey, or beef if you want to incorporate additional inexpensive proteins.
- **Don't Leave Your List:** Part of cooking at home should be meal planning (which we'll talk about below), and when you meal plan, you'll need to make a grocery list. Stick to your list as much as possible. Typically, it's the things you weren't planning to buy that somehow sneak into your cart and end up increasing your bill by twenty dollars.
- **Double Up:** Making big batches of food that can be eaten as leftovers for another meal or repurposed to create another dish will not only cut down on the time you spend cooking, it'll cut down on your bill, as you'll be buying fewer unique ingredients. This works particularly well with things like soups and casseroles, which aren't typically expensive in the first place and only taste better with time.

## Keep it Fun

Being in the kitchen doesn't have to feel like a casual trip to a torture chamber. If done right, it can be a great way to unwind and cap off the day on a healthy high note. Here are three ways to increase your enjoyment:

- **Team Up:** There's a reason why every rom-com features a kitchen scene where one person assembles a shitty pasta dish while the other awkwardly unbags a salad and drinks from a fishbowl of wine. No one really knows what that reason is, but cooking is indeed more fun with help. If you live with roommates, you can cook together or set up a rotating schedule where you each cook a meal once a week that feeds the whole house. Sharing a meal (and cleanup duties) with others is much more fun than cooking, eating, and doing dishes alone.

- **Distract Yourself:** Listen to a podcast, crank up some music, put on a movie in the background, or catch up with your parents on the phone while you cook. This is especially important if you don't enjoy cooking, as it will give you something else to look forward to.
- **Don't Bite Off More Than You Can Chew:** Don't plan to cook every single night. It's not realistic from a time or energy standpoint. Start with two meals a week that will provide you with leftovers and plan for inexpensive and relatively healthy "no-cook" nights in between with things like a bagged salad or a turkey sandwich. If you can tolerate slurping your dinner or you don't have teeth, soup is another option.

*"On Sundays, I would make big batches of roasted vegetables, pasta, soup, etc. that I knew were good quality and could be quickly warmed up while in a hurry. I would also precut fruit, make granola, and blend smoothies to have on hand for early mornings."*

—THE NEW SCHOOL, RECENT GRAD

## Tips for Sticking with It

Cooking is one of those adult responsibilities that can become a real pain in the ass if not tackled properly. Here are two additional ways to lessen that pain:

- **Meal Plan:** Spend time brainstorming your menu for the week. I usually do this on Sunday, but if you hate interrupting your weekend with something that feels like work, save it for Monday. That said, if you're only cooking a couple of meals, this shouldn't take more than five minutes. Figure out when and what you will cook, make a grocery list, and then go shopping for the ingredients ahead of time. Don't fight your schedule. Creating a realistic plan for the week should be based on which day you can go grocery shopping, and which nights will you have time to cook. Your "no-cook" or leftover dinners should occur on your busiest days. If you have the money, try a meal kit service. Though pricier than buying everything on your own, it removes the burden of shopping and planning.

*"Something that I have found really helpful is meal planning. I think of a couple different easy meals that I am excited about eating and plan them out each week."*
—CHAPMAN UNIVERSITY, SOPHOMORE

- **Food Prep:** Prepare for the upcoming week over the weekend, so that you've always got healthy options at the ready. Slice raw veggies, hard-boil eggs, make healthy muffins, bake sweet potatoes—you get the idea. These can be planned additions to your dinners, snack options, or full meals for breakfast or lunch. Prepping food for the week does not need to be a time-consuming or labor-intensive process, but a little work done on the front end will pay off when things get hectic during the week. Here's a tip: Save glass jars from jam, spaghetti sauce, and honey. They're easy to clean and the perfect size for storing things like smoothies, overnight oats, and veggies. Also, buy "ready-to-go" vegetables (like baby carrots, tiny cucumbers, and mini bell peppers) and fruits (like berries, apples, bananas). All of these make great snacks or additions to meals and don't require any prep work.

## The Struggle Is Real

Food is an emotionally complex component of the health equation. Discussions about what to eat can be charged and polarizing, similar to those about religion or politics. On one hand, food is fuel used to power the body, but on the other, it also provides comfort and happiness. Yet the best fuel isn't often what people associate with pleasure. When you don't know better, you just eat what's fun, but if you read the wrong advice, then you begin to believe that food shouldn't be fun at all. It's complicated and confusing and can surprise you by being one of the hardest parts of college and adult life to navigate.

I didn't know much about food before I got to college. My parents did all of the cooking at home, and I just ate whatever they made, most of which was healthy. You'd think that would have made it easier for me to make good choices once I was on my own, but that's not how it worked. Instead, I found myself surrounded by foods that I rarely had access to with no one to prevent me from eating as much of them as I wanted. I renamed the dining hall *Jilly: Unleashed*. Every day was cheat day during my first semester. The sheer abundance of choices was delightful: pancakes, bacon, tots for breakfast. Sandwiches for lunch. Pizza, burgers, fries for dinner. Cereal all the time, sometimes with chocolate milk just because I *could*. Soft serve after every meal. Easy Mac, ramen, and chips in my dorm room. I wolfed it all without an ounce of concern for my health.

I didn't realize I had gained weight until my grandma did a double take when she saw me at Christmas. "Wow, Jill, you look . . . *different*." By then, I had put on twenty pounds without noticing. However, neither her comment nor my newly skintight pants were enough motivation for me to change my eating or exercise habits. I liked my freedom, and I wasn't worried about my weight or my health.

During the summer between my sophomore and junior years, however, an asshole trainer at my internship glanced at my *wrist* and told me I was "big-boned." The body confidence or, frankly, body indifference that I had the luxury of experiencing up until that point in my life was gone in an instant, replaced by an acute awareness of how I looked in the mirror. I initially moved in the right direction by adding regular exercise to my life for the first time since high school. Unfortunately, I also started using a scale, which, coupled with my new negative body image, was the kiss of death. The exercise caused my body to change and made me feel confident and strong, but the scale made it about numbers. I liked losing weight. Dropping pounds helped me feel better about my body, but it escalated quickly. When I returned to school for my junior year, I eagerly started doing Weight Watchers with my two roommates.

*"The hardest adjustment was the food freedom. It was like being a kid in a candy store with unlimited money. I could try anything I wanted, and there were so many options."*
—MASSACHUSETTS INSTITUTE OF TECHNOLOGY, RECENT GRAD

The basic principle of Weight Watchers is to hit point allowance each day. I figured I'd lose more weight by coming in below that number, so I found ways to achieve that, such as working out to raise my point allowance and eating only low-calorie foods so that the impact on my daily total was minimal. On average, I was consuming 1,300 calories a day and burning around 400 at the gym.

In a matter of months, I lost twenty-five pounds. Everything I had gained and then some. At that point, things were out of hand. My previous lack of concern for what I was eating had shifted to the other extreme of unhealthy. My relationship with food had become dangerous. I was starving myself.

*"Many of my friends struggle with overexercising and negative self-image, and are completely preoccupied with what they eat."*
—SANTA CLARA UNIVERSITY, FRESHMAN

The convergence of several specific factors—namely increased stress, lack of structure, and heightened social pressures—make college the perfect breeding ground for eating disorders.[21] Students who grapple with anxiety are at the highest risk, though it can happen to anyone. According to the National Eating Disorders Association (NEDA), eating disorders typically emerge between the ages of eighteen and twenty-one. It's not a coincidence that this overlaps with college, as eating disorders tend to develop when the need to control an out-of-control environment becomes paramount.[22]

My roommates expressed their concern right around the time I was experiencing an extreme decrease in energy during exercise. I could barely make it through my workouts. It wasn't easy to admit, but deep down I knew that I needed to change my attitude toward food drastically. I talked to friends who'd had similar struggles. I got rid of the scale. I started learning about how to eat and care for myself the *right way*. Instead of fixating on a number and being led by a diet, I began listening to my body and focusing on eating well for my health. Over time, the question of "How do I look?" was replaced by "How do I feel?"

My story could have had a much different ending. It does for many. Thirty-five percent of students who experiment with dieting or food restrictions during college will end up becoming compulsive dieters. Of those, a quarter will end up with full-blown eating disorders.[23] According to a 2013 NEDA study, around 32 percent of college women and 25 percent of college men will struggle with an eating disorder—these numbers represent a more than 10 percent increase from a study done in 2000.[24]

The world of eating issues has a wide spectrum. What I struggled with is commonly referred to as "disordered eating," which itself encompasses quite a bit, from subscribing to fad diets and eating "clean" through vigilant restrictions, all the way up to binging and purging. The following is a short list of general symptoms for a broad range of disorders:[25,26]

- Preoccupation with weight, food, and calories
- Relentless pursuit of thinness
- Refusal to eat certain foods or food groups
- Engagement in food rituals
- Extreme concern with or distortion of appearance and body image
- Eating alone or in secret to avoid shame, guilt, or embarrassment
- Eating past the point of comfort
- Skipping meals or eating tiny portions
- Noticeable fluctuations in weight and swings in mood
- Feeling weak, faint, or dizzy
- Stomach cramps or pains
- Missing or having very irregular periods

If you are experiencing any of these symptoms, it might be worth consulting the screening tool on the NEDA website for a more thorough analysis of your behaviors. It may also be time to search for a specialist. Opening yourself up to help isn't always easy, but acknowledging that you need guidance is a great first step. *Everything* will get easier once you get started. You're not alone in this. There are people on your campus to help you understand what you're dealing with and to give you support the way you need it.

*"I didn't feel like I was good at anything freshman year. I went from a very small school to a very big school, so I didn't feel particularly 'special.' I realized one day that I could go all day without eating, and for some reason, I thought, Oh wow, this is cool. This is MY thing. I was going to be super into skipping meals. I started keeping this tally of how many meals I would skip a day and try to get at least two tallies a day. I think it's truly one of the dumbest things I've ever done. I was so lucky that it only lasted for about three months, and that it never developed into a more serious eating disorder. It stopped because I told someone from home about it, and they encouraged me to get help, which I did."*

—NEW YORK UNIVERSITY, RECENT GRAD

When I was struggling with my eating, food was a tremendous source of stress. It brought me no joy. Every decision at every meal felt like a test. Every bite that wasn't perfect was an opportunity to feel bad about myself. Ironically, food wasn't my issue—mindset was. Creating a positive relationship with food required an entirely new attitude.

For starters, I stopped shit-talking myself. I allowed myself to be honest about my choices without judgment. Instead of feeling terrible after eating something I "shouldn't have," I'd own that I ate something that didn't make me feel great physically and make a better choice the next time I grabbed food. It was an enormous relief to quiet the inner judgment. To just listen to my body and give myself freedom with choices while still being honest and holding myself accountable. Then I started to embrace the notion that some of what I ate needed to be fun! That food could still provide the same comfort and joy that it had back when I ate *everything* I wanted, so long as I mostly attempted to make good choices. The shift didn't happen overnight. It took a whole lot of time, effort, and guidance from others for me to get to a good place with food. However, the more I practiced tuning in to how I felt after eating and striving for the goal of feeling good both mentally and physically, the easier it became to allow myself choice without guilt and balance without restriction.

Finding a balance is possible for everyone, but there's no quick fix. There's no thirty-day plan. As silly as it sounds, learning *how* to eat well takes practice.

And that's okay! You'll have multiple opportunities every day to work at it. After all, you're trying to establish a healthy lifelong relationship with food. One that is both satisfying and nourishing. Please, *please* be kind to yourself during the process, as you won't figure it out all at once, and internal shit-talk is never helpful.

---

**How to Have the Talk.** My roommates' thoughtful way of expressing concern prompted me to examine my habits. If you find yourself in a situation where you are worried about a friend, talk to them. Tell them gently that you're concerned, ask them questions, and then listen to what they have to say. You should never underestimate the impact that a simple conversation can have on someone who is struggling. The following pointers are according to the National Eating Disorders Association:

1. **Find a Private Space.** Plan to talk to your friend in a location where you can be alone. Having this conversation will be personal and difficult, and interruptions can both be uncomfortable and derail any progress.

2. **Focus on the Facts.** Give specific examples of the behaviors you've personally witnessed that have concerned you. Be thoughtful about your tone—you don't want to sound accusatory, as that can cause the other person to feel defensive.

3. **Don't Undermine the Problem.** Encouraging your friend to "just eat" oversimplifies the issue. Eating disorders are not a choice. It's okay to recognize that fact in your conversation, as it'll help remove any shame or stigmatization they feel. Someone who is experiencing symptoms often needs professional help to manage the problem.

4. **Be Prepared for Resistance.** Not everyone who needs help is ready for it. There's a chance that you will be met with anger and denial. Don't snap back, and don't judge it. Just let your friend know that you care about them and will be there when they're ready. At this point, however, it may be best to share your concern with someone else to widen the net of people who may be able to help.

---

Experiment. Change a few things, then move on to a few more when you're ready. Make a game out of eating one healthy meal a week. When that's easy, up it to twice a week. Before you know it, you'll be at once a day. When it comes to your health, progress is perfect. The wonderful thing about making progress with food is that all positive changes, no matter how small, will make a noticeable difference in regard to how you feel.

## For When You Forget

Because we all take a pizza-fries-burgers-and-cookies-only vacation from time to time. If you're ready for a reset, start here:

- **Eat More Fruits and Veggies.** Shoot for a cup of fruit at breakfast, and a cup of veggies at both lunch and dinner to hit the minimum CDC recommendation.
- **Cut Back on Added Sugar.** Stop regularly indulging in sugar-heavy break-fast foods (as those set you up for a day of struggle), and kick your daily soda, energy drink, or sugar-bomb latte habit. Eat sweets, but aim for only once a day with either a dessert at lunch or dinner.
- **Be Thoughtful About Portions.** Grains are usually the hardest to moderate, so keep in mind that a serving is about the size of your fist, which likely equates to one or two scoopfuls or about a quarter of your plate.
- **Stock Healthy Snacks in Your Room.** Snacking seems to be both most appealing and most mindless at night, but you're unlikely to go overboard with low-sugar, low-salt foods, like Cheerios, unsalted popcorn, yogurt, or apples and nut butter. Chances are good that you won't be craving those things in the first place and will skip what is likely an unnecessary late-night meal altogether as a result. That doesn't mean you shouldn't indulge when you feel like it! You'll constantly be surrounded by excellent garbage in the dining hall and elsewhere on campus, so when the need to eat something delicious and unhealthy strikes, simply do it there. Allow your room to be a temptation-free zone.

Try to remember:

- **If Eating Is Causing You to Stress, Take Notice.** This could be an early warning sign of an eating issue. Check out the NEDA website, speak to a trusted friend or family member, or look to your campus counseling center for guidance. Remember that eating issues typically emerge between the ages of eighteen and twenty-one and are most common in women. Be honest with yourself about your behavior. The sooner you can course-correct, the better your chances of avoiding a more significant issue.

- **Actively Work on Cultivating a Healthy Relationship with Food.** Approach food as something to be explored and enjoyed. Rather than attaching yourself to intense restrictions or the newest fad, stick to a few simple rules to eat in a way that both gives you energy and makes you happy. You're going to have access to an abundance of options in college. Notice which foods make you feel your best and eat those most frequently, but give yourself permission to indulge your cravings. After all, the ultimate goal is to feel great, both physically and mentally, after you eat. Developing the right relationship with food can take time, but keep at it. You're going to be throwing down multiple meals a day for the rest of your life, so put in the necessary effort to settle into eating habits that feel responsible, satisfying, and sustainable. It takes time, but be patient. You can do this.

# CHAPTER 3

# BOOZE

## DAVE

**Jill had a strange introduction to booze.** During a time when many of her high school peers had begun testing the alcohol waters, she opted to give it a try during a sleepover. She and a friend snuck a Smirnoff Ice each from her dad's beer fridge and took their first sips in unison. The sugary, prepackaged spiked soda was so repulsive, she instantly gagged and wheezed. Uncontrollable guttural noises escaped her mouth in a tirade of *bleh* and *ew*, while she stopped, dropped, and rolled on the floor to extinguish the poison fire. Her friend just calmly watched and pondered where the cooler kids were hanging out. Never one to give up easily, Jill figured she could disguise the taste by pouring it over a big bowl of vanilla ice cream. *So gross.* She labored through half of the fizzy soup with constipated facial expressions before ultimately pouring it down the drain. This was the last time *that* friend slept over, and also the last time Jill drank until college.

My experience was on the other end of the spectrum. I first tried alcohol in junior high, and within a few years, I procured an ID (that worked) and had become the poster child for reckless behavior. In high school, doing beer runs at parties had turned into somewhat of a part-time job, and I carried all of that energy past graduation and straight into my freshman year at a small school in rural Iowa. When I got to college, all of the other idiots gravitated toward each other like moths to a flame. It's like we could just sense it when we met each other, "oh yeah, this guy fuckin parties." There was no shortage of willing participants. Our campus was pretty much surrounded by cornfields and little else, which undoubtedly contributed to the popularity of sitting in a room playing drinking games. Within a week, I knew a roster of people who prioritized cheap beer as their most important expense.

*"The college culture here is to drink as much as possible, and it is something that new students especially do to fit in."*

—BOSTON UNIVERSITY, SENIOR

Drinking removes inhibitions. It can make you feel happy, relaxed, and more confident in uncomfortable situations. It's common in college for all of those reasons—55 percent of students drink at least once a month, making it the substance of choice by a landslide. By contrast, just over 20 percent of college students smoke pot, 13 percent use e-cigarettes, and about 10 percent use prescription drugs (without a prescription).[1] And it's no wonder, especially for freshmen. Trying to make new friends can be super awkward, and booze can help take the edge off. It's called "liquid courage" for a reason.

That said, alcohol is illegal for the majority of first- and second-year students, who are typically still under twenty-one. Still, regardless of where you go to school, you're going to have access to alcohol and parties in a different way than ever before. Before you try your first keg stand, you should know that alcohol is poison—literally. You can die from drinking too much of it at once. And thousands of people do, every single year, which is pretty crazy if you think about it. Legally sold diluted poison annually kills thousands because they don't know it's diluted poison! But we're not here to condemn it. Because alcohol is dangerous and habit-forming, we want to give you a thorough introduction, so you know how to handle yourself if you choose to drink.

In this chapter, I will share my experiences, along with those of current college students, to hopefully give you an idea of what to expect. We'll take a look at the different types of booze, what they do to your body, and how to utilize drinking strategies to avoid nasty hangovers that will make you want to put your head in a microwave. Or a bear trap. Seriously, you'll want to cancel your life and sleep for all of October. I'm gonna lay some science on you, but it's not going to feel like health class. We're going to explore what happens when you get drunk and talk about how to determine your limit, so you're not puking into the garbage. We'll also cover the scary shit that can happen from *overdoing* it with alcohol because alcohol is poison, and too much poison is a bad thing. With a better understanding of how booze will affect you, you can have a good time *and* avoid shitting your pants or making a fool of yourself.

## New Friends and New Surroundings

Despite our different experience levels with drinking before college, Jill and I found ourselves in similar booze-happy climates when we arrived at our respective schools. As two highly competitive people, we found ourselves playing a lot of drinking games. This resulted in a lot of binge drinking, which is just a fancy term for sucking down an excessive quantity of alcohol in a short period of time. About 40 percent of college students participate in binge drinking, a number that's stayed roughly the same since 1994.[2]

We all take cues from the people around us. Especially when we're in unfamiliar, highly stressful social situations—like the beginning of college—the herd mentality gives us basic guidelines for how to act. *Everyone is on their phone. I'm gonna pull out my phone.* Observing the behavior modeled by others, accepting it as normal, and then imitating it is actually a form of peer pressure.[3] Though indirect, it can have a pretty serious effect on your choices by shaping the way you think. When it comes to alcohol, this is especially true at schools with high levels of binge drinking.

The first six weeks of college are a critical adjustment period that can easily be sabotaged by reckless drinking. If the social environment on your campus treats binge drinking as the standard, then it's understandable to consider it normal when you get there. Pounding ridiculous amounts of booze is an easier choice to make when seemingly *everybody's* doing it, and you want to fit in.[4]

*"During zero week (right before classes start), there's almost always an ambulance outside one of the freshman dorms. New students don't understand their limits. They go too hard and end up needing to get their stomachs pumped. This happened to my roommate. He was hospitalized for two days."*

—UNIVERSITY OF CALIFORNIA, LOS ANGELES, FRESHMAN

Keep in mind that you don't have to drink. Not *everybody* does. About one-quarter of college students don't drink at all,[5] and at the end of the day, no one is going to really care what you decide to do. *If* someone truly gives you shit for turning down a drink, screw 'em! There are a whole lot of people in this world, and the ones that don't respect your choices aren't worth your time. You've got shit to do!

*"I was worried that I would get pressured into drinking too much or that not wanting to go to frat parties would stop me from finding friends. As it turns out, no one cares if you do or don't drink. No one has ever pressured me to drink more or anything like that."*

—WASHINGTON UNIVERSITY, FRESHMAN

It's also entirely possible to have a good time with people who are drinking, even if you're not. In fact, your friends will probably be grateful to always have a designated sober buddy around.

We're not suggesting that you can't drink during your time on campus. However, if you're going to partake, you should understand that the people you surround yourself with will likely rub off on you. Don't feel bad for a second about being picky with who you spend your time with. The guy chugging a big bottle of whiskey is maybe not the best choice for your drinking buddy. Drinking too much too fast can lead to some dark places, but first, let's take a look at what it actually does to the body.

## Drinking Like a Fish

Despite its widespread popularity, binge drinking isn't a great way to be introduced to alcohol. It's not just that you're drinking a lot, it's that you're drinking a lot *quickly*, and this presents a real challenge for your liver.

*"Catching up is always a bad idea. I once came late to a party and tried to quickly get on everyone else's level, just to end up barfing on a bus to a bowling alley."*

—UNIVERSITY OF NOTRE DAME, SENIOR

A quick anatomy lesson: alcohol is absorbed through the stomach and small intestine and processed by the liver. The liver's main job is to filter harmful materials (including booze) out of your system, but there's a limit on how much alcohol it can process at once, which means whatever it can't handle continues to circulate in your bloodstream, including through your brain and other vital organs.

Let's imagine that your liver is a noble samurai warrior. It dismantles alcohol at a relatively fixed rate, roughly one drink per hour. However, it Ginsu chops most efficiently when it's given the time to completely break down one drink before starting on another. When multiple drinks stack up in a queue waiting to be processed, the rate that the liver processes alcohol actually slows down. The samurai is not only fighting multiple drinks at once but is doing so with one hand tied behind its back. Not a fair fight. The dulling down of your liver's abilities has very real implications for how you feel. The effects you'd feel from three drinks are greatly amplified if consumed in thirty minutes versus over the course of three hours, all because your liver simply can't keep up.

*"I drank way too much one night my first semester of college. We started playing 'Never Have I Ever,' taking sips per loss, and I was drinking straight vodka. After the game, we started taking big shots. I remember taking three before everything went black. I came to four hours later on the bathroom floor with two friends watching me. I spent the next twelve hours moping around and throwing up. We estimated I had about sixteen drinks in four hours. Basically, I could have died. I never drank that much again."*

—UNIVERSITY OF ARIZONA, RECENT GRAD

Additionally, because you can drink alcohol faster than you can process it, not all of the effects of binge drinking will kick in immediately. It's like having an IV drip filled with booze attached to your arm—it will take a long time to move into and out of your system because it only drips so fast. The effects of drinking excessively can last hours, sometimes well into the next day, as the liver works overtime to cut through all the booze.

## Blacking Out

I can't tell you how many times my roommate asked first thing in the morning, "What the fuck happened last night?" When you binge drink, it's common to wake up the next day wondering how a stop sign wound up in your dorm room. Or a French bulldog. A third of college students report engaging in behavior while drinking that they later regretted.[6] While some of these nights can amount to funny stories with friends, others can be, frankly, a little scary.

Early in my freshman year, I had received warnings for some minor drinking-related offenses and was required to meet with the supervising resident advisor (RA) for all freshman dorms. I really respected her and appreciated the way she treated me. She talked to me like I was an adult, and that meant a lot. During the meeting, our conversation segued from a general "How are you adjusting?" to a specific "So . . . tell me what happened last Friday." I had no idea what she was talking about.

We paddled upstream together, swimming circles awkwardly around details of a broken mirror in a women's bathroom on a floor of a building clear on the other side of campus. I laughed off the tension, genuinely not connecting the relevance of the scene she described to our current conversation. I told her it sounded like an interesting story, but I wasn't sure how I could add to it. She asked me again, directly, if I wanted to talk to her about *what happened last Friday*. I smiled and apologized, explaining that as much as I wished I could help her out, she was talking to the wrong person. She closed the folder in front of her—"I guess we're done here"—and asked me to leave.

As I walked back to my room, there was something I couldn't shake. It was the look in her eye—like I'd kicked her dog, pissed on her flowers, or set her Christmas tree on fire. When I told her I didn't know anything about the broken mirror in the bathroom, it was like I slipped her a piece of paper that said, "Caution! The person handing you this is an asshole and shouldn't be trusted."

It was actually *that* look on her face, mild

*"My friends would recount something I had said or done the night before, and I couldn't remember doing it. My entire perception of the night was off, missing gaps here and there. It was super unsettling."*

—UNIVERSITY OF SOUTHERN CALIFORNIA, FRESHMAN

shock, and disappointment, that triggered my memory. The hallway was dark. It was late. I couldn't grasp moments before or after, but there was something oddly familiar about her being upset with me.

The next day, I received a letter of formal probation. Poring through the details of the report, it was as if each sentence sent fragments from a past life straight to my frontal lobe. I was with a friend in her room in a women's dorm. While using the communal bathroom on her floor, I discovered a mirror with large writing that stated, *"Football Players are Fucking Morons."* I broke the mirror partly because I was a football player, but mainly because I was a fucking moron. The supervising RA was called and arrived at the scene where I described to her what I had done and why. I even signed an incident report that night. Of course, all of these details were alarming and shameful. I'd invaded the privacy of my fellow students and compromised the sanctity of a safe space that was not meant for me. In the process, I'd destroyed property that did not belong to me, and not-so-ironically validated the message's observation. All of this made me feel terrible and embarrassed, but by far, the scariest thing was that I had no memory of it. I'd blacked out.

Blacking out is pretty scary. It's not like passing out, where you unexpectedly fall asleep. When you black out, you're still awake and functioning, but later you have no memory of what took place. It was once described to me as "the camera is on, but nobody pressed the record button." People who have blacked out are capable of walking, talking, even driving a car, or having sex.

> *"I slept with my friend's roommate and didn't realize it had happened until two days later."*
> —UNIVERSITY OF SOUTHERN CALIFORNIA, RECENT GRAD

The fact that you could have sex with someone and not even know it happened is really dangerous, but we'll talk more about consent later. For now, let's stick with blackouts: How do they happen? You're most likely to black out when there's a rapid increase in blood alcohol content (BAC) in your body. You've had too much, too fast, and your liver can't keep up with the number of drinks you're throwing back. A blackout can be "complete or partial, depending on the severity of memory impairment."[7] The night I broke a mirror in my friend's dorm, I had a partial blackout. Memories I had forgotten entirely resurfaced thanks to cues (the look on my RA's face and the report).

So why are blackouts so common, or rather, why is it so common to drink enough alcohol to black out? Frankly, because it feels good to drink . . . at least in the beginning. It starts light, warm, and fuzzy. Inhibitions lower, and your judgment starts to shift. You're feeling loose and having fun, so . . . sure, you'll have another. People around you continue drinking, so you continue drinking. Maybe someone suggests taking a shot. Before you know it, you've had more than you planned to.

*"There was a night I had maybe ten drinks in three hours. It was primarily liquor. Playing a drinking game is what made it turn into a bad night . . . throwing up and memory loss. I wasn't drinking for any bad reasons. I wasn't stressed out or pressured to drink. I was just having too much fun and lost track of how much I'd had."*

—COLLEGE OF WILLIAM AND MARY, JUNIOR

So, let's talk strategy. If you're going to drink, I'm sure you'd prefer to have a good time and call it a night in your dorm with friends instead of on the floor of your local jail's drunk tank. Trust me, it's a thing. They'll lock you (and the other jerks) in a windowless room with no clocks and give you a sticky plastic mat to "sleep" on as your buzz slowly transforms into a hangover. To avoid the serious consequences of overdoing it with alcohol, you have to understand what *too much* means for you.

*"The combination of frat parties and nearby bars with relaxed rules led to a lot of excessive drinking my freshman year. I blacked out regularly, which only happened once in high school. There were so many ways to get alcohol."*

—SOUTHERN METHODIST UNIVERSITY, RECENT GRAD

## Drinking Like a Responsible Land Mammal

You can measure how much alcohol is in your system with a tool called a Breathalyzer. It's basically part calculator and part space-kazoo-from-the-future that only requires you to blow into one end like you're putting out candles on the biggest birthday cake of your life. In return, you'll get a numeric value that's, essentially, a snapshot of your current buzz.

BAC, or blood alcohol content, is a measure of the percent of alcohol in your blood. A BAC of .08 means that .08 percent of a person's blood content is alcohol. So how many drinks does it take to blow a .08? How much time must pass before your BAC drops? What if I had two beers and a shot? What if I drank on an empty stomach? Let's take a look at a few different types of drinks, how much each one increases your BAC, and what physical side effects can be expected at different BAC levels.

---

**Legal Limits.** While a BAC of .08 puts you in the category of being legally impaired in the US, you can still be charged for driving drunk if your BAC is anywhere above .00 and the officer deems your behavior dangerous. Penalties vastly increase in many states for a BAC over .15 because they have the highest mortality rates of all driving accidents. The majority of these accidents happen between midnight and 3:00 a.m.

Biking instead? Know the laws in your state. Although most places consider "driving under the influence" to only apply to operators of vehicles with motors, twenty states classify a vehicle as anything that transports a person, which includes those modes of transportation powered by legs. Looking for more ways to lose money and risk some jail time? Don't act like a drunken asshole around cops (or anyone). You can get slapped with a public intoxication charge in some states for simply *appearing* drunk and destroying property or posing a threat to the safety of yourself or others while in public.

*"I did not begin drinking socially until after I graduated from college, but this never prevented me from going out and having fun at normal parties with those who did drink quite a lot. I didn't have a problem with other people drinking, so nobody had a problem with me! If anything, it helped keep us that much safer at the end of the night. On the flip side, you can really tell when someone in college jumps right into drinking and/or anxiety-reducing drugs as a replacement for social skills."*

—RHODE ISLAND SCHOOL OF DESIGN, RECENT GRAD

## Types of Booze

Booze comes in many different flavors, sizes, and strengths. The overarching categories are beer, liquor, and wine—each having a plethora of styles and subcategories. For our purposes, we're going to group them primarily based on their alcohol by volume, or ABV, which is a value you can find on the label that indicates what percentage of your drink is alcohol. Basically, how strong it is.

### *Beer*

Light beer is the most common drink you'll find in college, mainly because it's cheap. There are more than twenty different styles of beer, and new hybrids are being created all the time. Still, the overwhelmingly dominant style is the lager. At room temp, they can taste like a combination of sawdust and pond water, but if you keep them cold, they can be refreshingly light and crisp.

Light beer, and some ales, will hover around 5 percent ABV. A "standard drink," according to health professionals, is a 12-ounce beverage that's 5 percent ABV. If you drink three light beers, you've had three "drinks." Some states have laws that permit supermarkets and convenience stores to sell only low-point beer (around 3.2 percent ABV), so if you go to school in Kansas, Minnesota, Colorado, or Utah, that's a thing.

Other styles of beer, typically those that fall into the ale subset—think IPAs, pale ales, brown ales, porters, stouts—can have higher ABVs, primarily ranging from 7 to 10 percent. If you see the words "double," "triple," or "imperial" on a label, it's a hint that the ABV is higher than 5 percent. A few percentage points might not seem like a big deal, but when multiple drinks are involved, higher-ABV beers will kick your ass in a hurry. Three beers at 8.1 percent are equal to almost five "drinks."

## Mixed Drinks

Liquor on its own can taste like pure gasoline, so the logical solution to combat the gag-reflex-inducing symptoms is to combine it with a nonalcoholic "mixer." Mixers are often sugary to better disguise the liquor, so while soda and juice are common culprits, a mixer can really be anything or a combination of things, including water.

Mixed drinks are potentially dangerous because they can be extremely potent. They can contain up to two to three times the alcohol content of a standard drink. Given the taste-masking capabilities of a sugary mixer, it can be challenging to gauge how much alcohol you're consuming. When your drink tastes like melted candy and makes you want to furiously dance like the air puppet on top of a car dealership, it can be easy to overdo it.

*"My friends and I had these big glass boots that held about ten beers each. One night we decided to make jungle juice in them. We mixed Everclear, pineapple juice, and a little bit of an energy drink. I had more than half a boot, and it might have been the worst decision of my life. I thought I was pretty sober and then was like, oh . . . this is bad. We decided to go out that night, and as soon as I opened my dorm room door, I hit a black wall. I don't remember a single thing after that point. I was completely gone. I was only drinking for 45 minutes. It was way too much in way too little time."*
—FORDHAM UNIVERSITY, SOPHOMORE

Everclear, by the way, is *extremely* potent at 95 percent ABV. It's twice as strong as vodka and nineteen times stronger than Budweiser. It's so powerful, in fact, that it can fuel a gas-powered lawnmower. No, really, I've seen the video.

If someone makes or gives you a mixed drink, it's good to be leery, for a variety of reasons. Firstly, it could be spiked with something. Rohypnol, GHB, and Xanax are all substances that sick fucks slip into people's drinks without their consent. These drugs can render victims unconscious or cause memory blackouts, putting people at risk of sexual violence. A recent study that surveyed over six thousand college students from multiple universities found 7.8 percent of participants reporting that they had had their drinks spiked with illicit substances.[8] It does happen, so if someone you've never (or just) met comes up to you with a Solo cup, pass, and repeat after me: "Thanks, I'm good."

*"Our house's signature drink: 'Sorry Mom's.' A guaranteed hangover consisting of Mountain Dew and the cheapest rum available. This is one of the scariest drinks because you don't taste any alcohol going down. There is simply too much sugar."*

—SANTA CLARA UNIVERSITY, RECENT GRAD

Secondly, if someone else makes your drink, you may have no idea how much alcohol they poured in. For liquor, one "drink" is a shot glass worth of booze—the

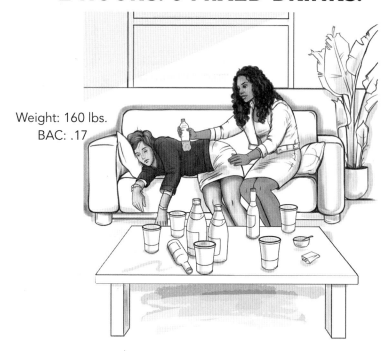

**2 HOURS. 3 MIXED DRINKS.**

Weight: 160 lbs.
BAC: .17

standard is 1.5 ounces of 40 percent ABV—but people regularly pour more than this when making a mixed drink. That fruity-sweet cup of jungle juice someone hands you could easily contain two or three "drinks" worth of alcohol. This makes it easy to get much drunker than you ever intended to, especially if you have multiple mixed drinks in a night.

Let's consider a scenario! Two women go to a party together, and one ends up downing three strong mixed drinks (the equivalent of six standard drinks) within a period of two hours. At 160 pounds, this takes her BAC all the way up to .17, and that's assuming she hadn't been drinking at all before she arrived.

Feelings of fun will be replaced with blurry vision, the spins, and the urge to puke. She may need some help getting home. She will likely wake up the next morning thinking, *How did I get so drunk last night? I only had a few drinks,* but given the BAC she climbed to, she may also find that she has holes in her memory. It's far too easy to drink way past your limit *by accident* with mixed drinks, which is why it's a good idea to stop yourself after one or avoid them altogether.

## Shots

Ever wonder why it's called a "shot?" There are many theories about its etymology, but let's keep it simple: go ahead and punch yourself in the face. That's what taking too many shots will feel like tomorrow. Fancy shots are typically mixtures of liquors (vodka, whiskey, tequila, etc.), liqueurs (sweetened liquors which are sometimes, but not always, less strong), and mixers. In contrast, straight shots are just pure poison.

*"I stopped doing shots after freshman year because I realized how much I didn't like them. There is a weird pressure to do shots because it is a communal activity, or to drink liquor in drinking games, but honestly nobody gives a shit if you don't actually take the shot."*

—OBERLIN COLLEGE, JUNIOR

Taking a shot is pretty much the fastest way to inject alcohol into your system because consumption is so immediate. One full drink (1.5 ounces of 40 percent ABV) in less than five seconds? You're literally pouring booze into your stomach, and all but guaranteeing a significant spike in your BAC. I recommend avoiding shots altogether, but if you're going to have a Slippery Nipple, Mind Eraser, or a Gorilla Crotch Punch, try limiting yourself to only one. They can be especially dangerous if you've already been drinking. When you're a little tipsy and someone orders a round of shots, you may think, *Why not?* Unfortunately, this type of instant injection of alcohol can be the difference between a good night and a bad one.

### Wine

If you're drinking wine in college, because you wear turtlenecks or watch *Real Housewives*, there are a few things that you should know. Wine is, on average, more than *two* times stronger than beer. There is a broad alcoholic spectrum available (5 percent to 20 percent), but the most common wines tend to fall in between 11 and 16 percent ABV. The American standard serving size is five ounces of 12 percent ABV.

# STANDARD SERVING SIZES

Two fingers below top for
**12 OZ OF BEER**

5% ABV or less
Keystone Light, Michelob Ultra, Coors Light, Yuengling, Corona, Pabst Blue Ribbon, Dos Equis, Miller High Life, Busch Light, Natural Light, Bud Light

Three fingers above bottom for
**5 OZ OF WINE**

12% ABV or less
Chardonnay, Pinot Grigio, Riesling, White Zinfandel
14% ABV or less
Cabernet Sauvignon, Merlot, Pinot Noir
**Lighter color = Lower ABV**
*ABV will differ by brand*

One finger above bottom for
**1.5 OZ OF LIQUOR**

40% ABV = 80 proof
Vodka, Tequila, Gin, Rum, Whiskey

*18 oz. plastic cup*

## Stages of Intoxication

Alcohol is not an on/off switch. The more you drink, the more intoxicated you'll become; and there is quite a spectrum of feelings, ranging from "warm and fuzzy" to "unable to move." The side effects experienced at certain BAC levels are well documented. They start out great and, frankly, slowly turn terrible with the more you drink. The stages of intoxication have quite an overlap—there isn't a clear graduation from one to the next. It's easiest to focus on where they begin and understand that the symptoms associated with each stage will eventually dissipate and be replaced with something worse. It's kind of like playing a video game where you're reincarnated after every level into something slower and more useless. You start as a human. By level three, you're a sloth. By level five, you're a stump that gets pissed on by all the neighborhood dogs. Anyway, here are the six stages of impairment:

1. **Mild Impairment: *Euphoria.*** A quick jolt of intense happiness is one of the first things you'll feel when drinking. It's awesome. By far, this is the best stage. It's the hook—a burst of life and possibility that eases tension and spurs laughter. You may find it easier to communicate and connect with others and may even feel a bit more courageous. Euphoria enters the equation after one standard drink, when you hit a BAC around .02 or .03. If you continue to drink, you will continue to feel euphoria—until it abandons you at .12 and is replaced by its evil twin, dysphoria. More on that son of a bitch later.

2. **Increased Impairment: *Excitement.*** Despite the name, this level does not mean you feel like it's Christmas morning. It means you're becoming emotionally unstable and (ironically) drowsy. You're also, by this point, experiencing a profound loss of coordination. If you've entered this realm, you are now legally intoxicated and have a BAC of .09 or above.[9] If you're in public with a BAC this high, you can be charged with—wait for it—public intoxication. Excitement lasts from .09 to .20, and it's during this stage that you will begin to experience memory loss (a blackout).

3. **Severe Impairment: *Confusion.*** Around .18, the blacked-out sloppy drunk becomes mentally confused.[10] Someone this drunk may not know where they are or what they are doing. A BAC this high only results from drinking excessively

in a short amount of time. Blackouts at this stage are highly likely. People this drunk can also be a little scary and have the potential to become emotional, aggressive, withdrawn, or overly affectionate. They will have trouble seeing and stagger. If you've ever heard of someone getting the "spins" —being so dizzy they have to lie down—they are in a state of drunken confusion. They may feel sleepy and slur their speech, and they may not feel pain like they do when they're sober. At this stage, there's an even more severe drop in coordination. If you threw anything to them, they certainly wouldn't catch it, and their reaction time would be so slow that it'd likely hit them before they had time to try.[11] I definitely wouldn't pick someone in this state to be on my dodgeball team.

> *"My best friend and I went to a party one night. I wasn't with her a lot of the time when she was taking shots, so I have no idea how many she took. Everything was fine, and then she couldn't stand up by herself. They tried to give her water, but she still looked very pale. I was a little out of it, trying to help where I could. She kept throwing up over and over again. She has no memory of it. One person suggested that we not send her to EMS. 'She's all right. This happens.' When another friend, who was more sober, asked what we should do, I was like, 'HELLO? We call the ambulance!' To think no one would have called. . . . My friend literally threw up at least twelve times. Her BAC was at .38."*
>
> —TUFTS UNIVERSITY, FRESHMAN

4.  **Severe Impairment: *Stupor.*** At this stage, things get very scary. A drunken stupor occurs between .25 and .4 and can be an indication of alcohol poisoning.[12] An individual with a BAC this high has effectively rendered the body incapable of clearing the toxins generated by alcohol metabolism. Remember the samurai warrior? He's long lost the battle by now. Someone this drunk will not be able to stand or walk, respond to stimuli, control bodily functions (i.e., they may piss or shit themselves), and they'll either be in a stupor or passed out. A person in a stupor is at very high risk for respiratory complications and choking on their own vomit. If you observe someone experiencing these symptoms, getting them medical assistance could save their life.

# EXPECTED IMPAIRMENT BASED ON BAC

| BAC RANGE | LEVEL OF MENTAL IMPAIRMENT self-control, judgment, reasoning, memory, assessment of danger | LEVEL OF PHYSICAL IMPAIRMENT balance, coordination, vision, speech, hearing, reaction time | OTHER NOTES | STAGE |
|---|---|---|---|---|
| .02 to .03 | Insignificant | Insignificant | Mildly relaxed. Loss of shyness. | LOW LEVEL INTOXICATION |
| .04 to .06 | Minor | Insignificant | Warm. Relaxed. Emotions heightened. | EUPHORIA |
| LEGALLY INTOXICATED AT .08 | | | | |
| .07 to .09 | Moderate | Minor | May believe impairment is less than it is. | |
| .10 to .125 | Significant | Moderate | Slurred speech. | EXCITMENT |
| .13 to .15 | Severe | Significant | Becoming anxious and restless. | |
| .16 to .19 | Severe | Severe | Vomiting possible. Will look visibly drunk. | CONFUSION |
| 0.20 | Severe | Severe | Blackouts and vomiting likely. | |
| 0.25 | Severe | Severe | Risk of choking on vomit or injury by falling. | DYSPHORIA |
| 0.30 | Severe | Severe | May pass out and be difficult to wake up. | STUPOR |
| 0.35 | Severe | Severe | Coma possible. | |
| 0.40 | Severe | Severe | Death possible. | |

5. **Life-Threatening Impairment: *Coma.*** *Holy shit.* Once your BAC climbs up to .35, things really take a turn for the worse. You have the potential to enter a coma. Your body's ability to breathe and circulate blood through all of your vital organs will become severely depressed. Motor response and reflexes will be negligible, and the body temperature will drop. Anyone with this much alcohol in their system is at risk of death.[13]

6. **Life-Threatening Impairment: *Death.*** When your BAC climbs above .40, you will stop breathing. It's hard to fathom how one could drink enough to reach this point, but it's a tragic reality that all comes back to the fact that alcohol takes time for your body to process. If you overload your system with too much booze at one time, your body simply can't keep up, and under extreme circumstances, it will shut down.

## The Tipping Point

There is a very specific BAC range that is a tipping point for positive and negative side effects—an easy-to-cross line that separates the good from the bad. When a person has a few drinks and becomes legally intoxicated (.08), they have experienced good feelings: euphoria, loss of shyness, relaxation. It's understandable for someone to connect these "good" feelings to the act of drinking, and to want to keep the train rolling because of that.

*"I drank eight shots of Everclear in the span of two hours. It was great. I got the full experience of having an ambulance called on me and a $310 medical bill."*

—UNIVERSITY OF ROCHESTER, FRESHMAN

However, drinking more alcohol when you're already intoxicated brings you closer to the dark side. Around .12, euphoria's evil twin comes a-callin'. Dysphoria. *Dun dun dun!*

Dysphoria is a state of unease, anxiety, restlessness, and general dissatisfaction that kicks into effect as your BAC rises above .12 and intensifies the drunker you get. A person experiencing dysphoria shows signs of being a "sloppy" drunk. Blurred vision with significant loss of balance, gross motor impairment, and a lack of physical control. They may seem unreasonably irritable. You can pretty quickly identify people this intoxicated by the way they slur their speech. They may also have

bloodshot eyes and a distant gaze. Their vision, hearing, and (maybe most importantly) judgment will be impaired. The odds of them acting like an asshole increase
by about 5,000 percent. At this point, the soft and hazy dreamlike state of being
drunk begins to turn into a nightmare.

You never need to go past 0.12. EVER. *This is your ceiling.* The limit. The point
where you need to cut yourself off. Commit this number to memory. We're going
to give you the tools to calculate just how many drinks this means for you, but first,
we need you to answer a few questions about yourself.

## Alcohol and You

A handful of factors make up how you will respond to alcohol. Here are the four
most important things to consider:

- **Your Sex and Weight.** Let's start with a scenario. A 180-pound man and
  a 140-pound woman pregame at a friend's house. Both have four drinks
  worth of alcohol over an hour and decide to hit the road. Though they've
  had the same amount to drink in the same amount of time, they are having vastly different experiences. Her BAC level is almost double his. She
  will look drunk, slurring her speech, and struggling to walk without losing
  her balance. She will also have a delayed reaction time, a lack of coordination, and an inability to track moving objects. Feelings of nausea aren't
  far off. Simply put, she is trashed. He, on the other hand, is feeling warm,
  fuzzy, and funny. He's got a big dopey smile on his face and is relaxed and
  happy. While he definitely shouldn't drive a car because his judgment and
  reaction time are slightly impaired, he still has relatively good control over
  his body.

    Yes, alcohol affects men and women differently, and it all revolves
  around water. In general, women tend to have a higher percentage of body
  fat than men. Fat tissue contains less water than lean tissue, so the average man is made up of 60 percent water. In contrast, the average woman
  consists of 55 percent water. The slight difference in the total amount of
  water means that the concentration of any amount of alcohol in a woman's

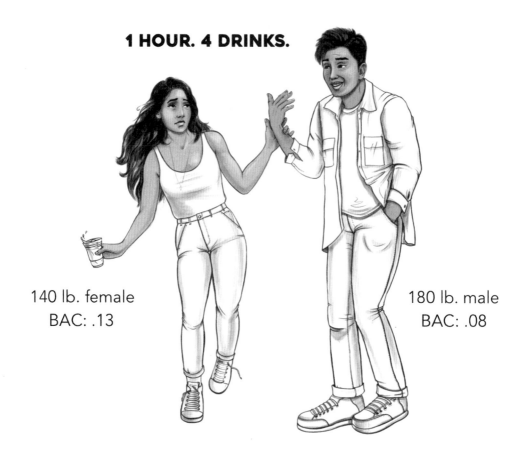

**1 HOUR. 4 DRINKS.**

140 lb. female
BAC: .13

180 lb. male
BAC: .08

system would be higher than if the same amount of alcohol was added to a man's system. Thus, women achieve higher BAC levels after drinking equivalent amounts of alcohol.[14,15] If a woman and a man are the same weight, the difference is relatively minor, but discrepancies really show up with two opposite-sex drinkers of different sizes. Bottom line: don't go drink for drink with someone who's playing in a different category. The outcomes won't be comparable.

- **Hungry or Full?** Drinking on an empty stomach is a bad idea, and it all has to do with the way your body absorbs alcohol, and more specifically, *where* the action happens. While your stomach does absorb some of the booze into your blood (up to 20 percent), the vast majority of the absorbtion takes place in your small intestine (more than 75 percent).[16] This means if your stomach is empty, the alcohol passes right into your small intestine where it rapidly enters your blood, quickly spikes your BAC, and greatly increases your chances of experiencing negative side effects. If your stomach is full, the drinks will hang out for their own little digestion dance party, moving on over time, and lowering the risk of wanting to puke your guts out.

- **Body Type.** The way you're built also plays a part in how booze will impact you. An overweight person will be more affected than a lean, muscular one, and again, it's all due to the amount of water in your body. I'm not talking about how much water you drink; I mean on a cellular level, a lean person is comprised of more water than an overweight person because fat tissue contains less water than lean tissue. More fat tissue means less body fluids and, ultimately, a higher concentration of alcohol in the blood. There are also special considerations for certain ethnicities. Some people of Asian heritage, mainly Chinese and Japanese, have fewer enzymes that break down alcohol.[17] People who carry this gene may feel drunker faster than people who don't have it.

- **Drinking History.** Your experience plays a large part in how alcohol affects you. The more frequently a person drinks, the higher their tolerance for alcohol will become. They need to drink more than they used to in order to achieve the same desired effect.[18] However, this does not mean that a person with a high tolerance processes alcohol faster. The amount of alcohol you put in your system will be accurately reflected in your BAC, *regardless of tolerance*. In other words, if drinking two beers in half an hour raises your BAC to .08 as a new drinker with a low tolerance, it will also raise your BAC to .08 if you become a heavy drinker with a high tolerance. Building up a high tolerance does not give you an advantage. On the contrary, having a high tolerance increases the likelihood of unintentionally overconsuming and sending your BAC dangerously high.

## Finding Your Limit

We've finally made it to the fun part—*charts!* While the formula for *how* alcohol will affect you is mildly complex, the measurement for *how much* alcohol is in your body is exact. Assuming similar tolerance levels, a small woman with a BAC of .08 will feel basically the same thing as a large man with a BAC of .08—what differs is the amount each of them would have to drink in order to reach that BAC. John (240 pounds) will reach .08 after having five drinks over forty-five minutes. Jane reached .08 somewhere shortly after her second drink. *Big difference.*

*"I've found a rule of thumb that works for me: I won't have more than two or three drinks on a night, and I stick to that. It's worked out well thus far because I like to drink, but I want to stay within my bandwidth of control and cognition. Plus, waking up late and feeling hungover the next day is such a waste."*

—UNIVERSITY OF SOUTHERN CALIFORNIA, SENIOR

Using your sex, weight, and approximate length of time you will be drinking, you can estimate your BAC for different scenarios. You can use charts like the one on the next page to set your intention for any given night, but more importantly, to figure out the number of drinks you should never surpass. Understand that these BAC values are only approximations, as the factors we just talked about (body type, food, and drinking history) will also affect you. Something to keep in mind is that our bodies can process between .015 percent and .020 percent of alcohol every hour (about one drink for most people), so you can subtract .015 off the BACs given to adjust for specific durations of consumption. For the most part, the potential for fun is greatest between a BAC of .02 and .08, but shit gets super unpleasant after .12. In case it's not clear yet, you *never* need to drink enough to send your BAC above .12. Think of this as your ceiling, your max, your drink limit for the night. Use the estimated BAC chart to determine how many drinks you can have before you should call it quits, and notice that this changes over time. Your body *does* process alcohol at a rate of about one drink per hour, so the longer you're out, the more alcohol your body can break down. And by the way, you don't need to drink to your ceiling every time. It's not a target, but rather a cutoff point. Go find your maximum

# ESTIMATED BAC

## WOMEN

| Drinks | Weight (lbs.) | | | | | | | |
|---|---|---|---|---|---|---|---|---|
| | 100 | 120 | 140 | 160 | 180 | 200 | 220 | 240 |
| 1 | .05 | .04 | .03 | .03 | .03 | .02 | .02 | .02 |
| 2 | .09 | .08 | .07 | .06 | .05 | .05 | .04 | .04 |
| 3 | .14 | .11 | .10 | .09 | .08 | .07 | .06 | .06 |
| 4 | .18 | .15 | .13 | .11 | .10 | .09 | .08 | .08 |
| 5 | .23 | .19 | .16 | .14 | .13 | .11 | .10 | .09 |
| 6 | .27 | .23 | .19 | .17 | .15 | .14 | .12 | .11 |
| 7 | .32 | .27 | .23 | .20 | .18 | .16 | .14 | .13 |
| 8 | .36 | .30 | .26 | .23 | .20 | .18 | .17 | .15 |
| 9 | .41 | .34 | .29 | .26 | .23 | .20 | .19 | .17 |
| 10 | .45 | .38 | .32 | .28 | .25 | .23 | .21 | .19 |

## MEN

| Drinks | 120 | 140 | 160 | 180 | 200 | 220 | 240 | 260 |
|---|---|---|---|---|---|---|---|---|
| 1 | .03 | .03 | .02 | .02 | .02 | .02 | .02 | .01 |
| 2 | .06 | .05 | .05 | .04 | .04 | .03 | .03 | .02 |
| 3 | .09 | .08 | .07 | .06 | .06 | .05 | .05 | .04 |
| 4 | .12 | .11 | .09 | .08 | .08 | .07 | .06 | .06 |
| 5 | .16 | .13 | .12 | .11 | .09 | .09 | .08 | .08 |
| 6 | .19 | .16 | .14 | .13 | .11 | .10 | .09 | .09 |
| 7 | .22 | .19 | .16 | .15 | .13 | .12 | .11 | .11 |
| 8 | .25 | .21 | .19 | .17 | .15 | .14 | .12 | .12 |
| 9 | .28 | .24 | 0.21 | .19 | .17 | .15 | .14 | .14 |
| 10 | .31 | .27 | .23 | .21 | .19 | .17 | .15 | .15 |
| 11 | .34 | .32 | .25 | .23 | .21 | .19 | .17 | .17 |
| 12 | .37 | .35 | .28 | .25 | .23 | .20 | .19 | .19 |

### SUBTRACT .015 FOR EVERY HOUR ELAPSED SINCE FIRST DRINK

| Hrs | 1 | 2 | 3 | 4 | 5 | 6 | 7 | 8 |
|---|---|---|---|---|---|---|---|---|
| Subtract | .015 | .03 | .045 | .06 | .075 | .09 | .105 | .12 |

Ex: Estimated BAC for a 140 lb. female who consumes 4 drinks over 4 hours = .13 - .06 = .07
Estimated BAC for a 180 lb. male who consumes 8 drinks over 4 hours = .17 - .06 = .11

drink limit right now. Commit it to memory. Write it down on your hand, tattoo it on your wrist, put a Post-it note on your fridge. Your ceiling is arguably the most important thing to know if you're going to be drinking.

## How to Drink

Time for an action plan! Getting absolutely wasted can be really dangerous, so don't put yourself in that position. I promise, you can still have all of the fun while staying safe, and ideally not be hungover and worthless the next day. All it takes is a plan. Here are seven components to keep in mind:

1. **Set Your Limit.** Staying in the BAC sweet spot (.02 to .09) increases the odds that you'll have a fun, puke-free night, so figure out how many drinks it'll take for you to get there by using the BAC table. This should be a part of your evening plan, right next to with whom and how are you getting home.

    *"I like the drinking environment and drink one to three times per week, but I do not like being hungover. I've learned that three drinks is my limit so that I can function the next day."*
    —COLLEGE OF WILLIAM AND MARY, JUNIOR

    Additionally, set your limit for the week. How many days do you want to go out? Determine when you need to take care of business and when you can let loose. This will give you a better balance between schoolwork and hanging out with friends. It also allows you to plan what nights you can devote to taking care of yourself in ways that don't involve alcohol. Maybe this is when you work out, see live music, or just do laundry.

2. **Know How Many *Drinks* Are in Your Drink.** It can be tricky to look at one heavily poured shot and realize that there are TWO drinks in it. *But it's so small!?* Remember that the standard for a drink is a 12-ounce beer (at 5 percent ABV), a 5-ounce glass of wine, or 1.5 ounces of hard liquor. Mixed drinks can hold upward of three drinks of alcohol in one single cup. If that's the case, you should probably be done for the night after one of those. Be mindful of how much alcohol is in your cup. Always mix your own drink at a party, or at least watch your drink being mixed so you can judge how strong it is.

3. **Do Not Drink on an Empty Stomach.** Eat something before you go out. If you're about to start drinking and you haven't eaten in a while, make it your mission to find food. Why put yourself in a situation where you're riding the vomit comet and hugging a toilet all night?

> *"I never drank before college and didn't know my limits, which led to a few incidents of throwing up and bad hangovers the next day. After fall quarter, I stopped taking shots. I also make an effort now to sip drinks over a longer period of time, and I carry around a cup of water in between drinks. It helps me be conscious of how much I'm drinking, and no one knows the difference."*
> —UNIVERSITY OF CALIFORNIA, LOS ANGELES, FRESHMAN

4. **Drink Water.** The best cure for a hangover actually takes place *while* you're drinking. Drink a glass of water after each alcoholic drink. This will not only help combat the dehydrating effects of alcohol, but it will also increase the time in between drinks. If you're pregaming in a dorm room or at a house party, bring a bottle of water with you. When people overdo it with booze, it's because they drink too much, too fast—so don't drink too fast. By spacing out your drinks with water in between, you reduce the painful side effects that you'll experience in the morning. This is easy to do while pregaming but gets harder to maintain after you go out. If you're at a bar, order yourself a water or club soda with lime if you want it to look like a drink. If you're going out to party on campus, bring a small plastic bottle you can throw away, or fill up your cup with some water from the tap.

5. **Use the Buddy System.** Even though you're not on a field trip to the zoo, it's still good to have someone looking out for you. As the night gets later and people inevitably scatter, avoid situations where you are left by yourself. Especially for women, being alone late at night around intoxicated

> *"Always make sure you have at least one person who has your back when you go drinking."*
> —NEW YORK UNIVERSITY, RECENT GRAD

people makes you a target. It's so sad that *this* is a problem, but it is, and it's important to protect yourself. So when you're going out, make sure you've got someone to go with.

6. **Do Not Drive.** The most dangerous thing a drunk person can do is drive a car. Almost two thousand college students die per year from alcohol-related injuries, the vast majority of which come from motor-vehicle crashes.[19] Some studies have found that a quarter of all college students have driven under the influence.[20] There are so many dire risks—hurting yourself, hurting others, getting a DUI—it's just never fucking worth it. Always make a plan about how you're getting home *before* you leave for the night so that you're not relying on the judgment-impaired version of yourself to figure it out. Take an Uber or Lyft, call a taxi, or go out with a designated driver.

Speaking of drivers—don't get into a car with a driver who has been drinking. According to the College Alcohol Study (CAS) conducted by the Harvard School of Public Health, 23 percent of college students said they'd ridden with a driver who was high or intoxicated.[21] If your designated driver decided to have a few drinks after all, *don't get in their car*. Changing your plan when you have a feeling that you're putting yourself in a dangerous situation is the right thing to do. Again, don't get into the car with someone who is fucked up. The consequences can cost you your life.

Even when you are the designated sober driver (or riding with one), the roads can be precarious late at night. Two-thirds of all alcohol-related fatalities involving a car happen between midnight and 3:00 a.m.[22] The best way to ensure your safety is to be aware of your environment—not just *where* you are, but *who* you are around.

*"We were [driving] to a party and following a friend because we didn't know the way. The person we were following was driving crazy, driving on the line of the highway. We didn't know whether he was changing lanes or just playing around. Then, going around a sharp bend, he turned on two wheels and lost control and crashed into another car. The driver was drunk, and four of my friends were hospitalized."*

—COLLEGE ALCOHOL STUDY[23]

**For When You Turn Twenty-One.** On the day that you finally reach the legal drinking age, everyone will encourage you to go big. You will likely receive free drinks, either from mischievous friends or generous bartenders. It's easy to get carried away.

Bradley McCue was a junior at Michigan State University when he went out with friends to celebrate his twenty-first birthday. It was a common tradition on campus to "drink your age," and so Brad had proceeded to take twenty-one shots. Not to be outdone by a buddy's personal record of twenty-three, Brad took three more shots and called it a night. All of this drinking took place over ninety minutes. His friends helped him get home and safely into bed. His BAC reached .44, and the coroner estimated that he stopped breathing around 4:30 a.m. Brad died on his birthday. The official autopsy read, "This 21-year-old man died of ethanol poisoning, as a consequence of consuming a large amount of alcoholic beverage within a short period of time."[24]

Please take the time to visit Brad21.org and help his loved ones continue to spread awareness through his story. They've collected a plethora of invaluable resources with the mission of "encouraging and enabling responsible decisions" concerning alcohol.

*"Be leery of twenty-first birthdays. It normally starts off with a couple of beers or cocktails, and then on to shots at the bars. Barhopping probably starts around 10:00 p.m., and you're done around 1:00 a.m. Sometimes the birthday person can't even walk straight at that point."*

—UNIVERSITY OF ARIZONA, RECENT GRAD

## On a Lighter Note

We're going to continue our detour from darkness to talk about calories and then hangovers. *Fun!* I know. We're the worst.

### Booze Makes You Fat

I cannot count the number of burritos I have destroyed in a feverish bout of drunk munchies. I've made an entire pizza disappear countless times, and I've been so focused on food fulfillment missions that I've walked miles for it. *Miles.* Street hot dogs, frozen yogurt, fast food—honestly, anything. I had no real concept or concern for calories or contents. As Jill mentioned in the food chapter, there are some strategies you can employ to make sure you don't go overboard with these meals, but even if you choose to, at least now you know what you're getting yourself into. The drunk munchies were a meal I planned for and expected—one that I knew wasn't going to be healthy. But what I didn't understand was the enormous number of calories I'd been consuming from the booze itself. Entire meals' worth of calories, and in some cases, whole *days'* worth of calories. I was completely oblivious.

*"I gained seven pounds between winter break and spring break my Freshman year. I believe late-night munchies contributed, but more so, the alcohol. I think most students drastically increase their alcohol intake in college and don't realize the weight gaining consequences."*

—SCRIPPS COLLEGE, FRESHMAN

If you don't know how many calories are in your favorite booze, you're not alone. A study in 2008 found that two out of three college freshmen had no idea how many calories common alcoholic drinks contained.[25] There is a fantastic reason for this: nutrition labels are not required on alcoholic beverages, which makes no sense whatsoever!

Nutrition labels are required on almost all packaged food, even bottled water. *Bottled water!* There are seventeen zeros on the nutrition label for bottled water because it's NOTHING. BUT. WATER. However, if a product contains alcohol, no nutritional information is needed.[26] This is crazy considering when you buy a bottle of lemonade, the manufacturer is required by law to tell you the serving size and servings per container, as well as a breakdown of calories, sugar, fats, and cholesterol. However, if you buy a bottle of lemonade that contains alcohol, like Mike's Hard Lemonade, none of this information is provided. It has 390 calories, by the way—about the same number as a cheeseburger. *Let that sink in for a second.*

If you have multiple drinks in a night, the calories can add up quickly. To use the example above, three Mike's Hard Lemonades contain 1,170 calories. That's almost six Snickers bars and not the bite-size kind. You'd have to run twelve miles to burn this many calories, or do 3,900 sit-ups, or 5,500 jumping jacks, and let's be honest, you're not going to do that with a hangover. A night of heavy drinking can easily provide more calories than eating a fourth meal. Not all alcoholic beverages are this high calorie; both light beer and vodka shots are closer to 100 calories per serving. If you have a go-to drink that's not featured here, google the calorie content. There's lots of information online.

*"Most people don't understand that alcohol has SO many calories. You think of a shot as a quick thing that is gone in a second, but don't even consider the calorie deposit. I assumed beer was really high-caloric because of the term 'beer guts,' but I never applied the same logic to liquor or wine."*
—UNIVERSITY OF CALIFORNIA, LOS ANGELES, FRESHMAN

## Frat Boy Connor's Thirsty Thursday

So how many calories could you consume on a gluttonous rampage? Let's take a look at the toll a bingy night can take on the body. One thing you'll quickly discover in college is that the weekend starts on Thursday night. One such Thursday, our fictional hero—let's call him Frat Boy Connor—pregames in his buddy Crazy Dave's dorm room starting at 8:00 p.m. He ate two custom burgers and fries at the dining hall two and a half hours prior. Connor, who weighs 180 pounds, crushes five beers while playing drinking games, and splits a party-size bag of chips with a few other people. At 10:00 p.m., Connor and his friends head to the bars, taking a shot of whiskey on their way out the door. He stays at the bar from 10:30 p.m. to 1:00 a.m., consuming two heavily poured whiskey Cokes. He has one more pint of beer to close out the night and grabs a Hot-n-Ready pizza from Little Caesars with two sides of ranch dressing on the way home.

> *"Since my freshman year, I've definitely cut down on drinking. My classes have become harder, and I'm trying to stay healthy. I now go out once a week instead of multiple times a week. Also, surrounding myself with people who model a healthy lifestyle has encouraged me to become healthier."*
>
> —TULANE UNIVERSITY, JUNIOR

So what can we gather from Connor's evening of indulgence? For starters, holy shit, that's a lot of calories. The average man only needs 2,500 calories a day. *For a full day.* I hope he brought his comfortable shoes because to burn off 5,305 calories on a treadmill, Connor's going to need to run fifty miles. But that's assuming Connor even remembers everything that he ate. At a BAC of .173, he reached blackout territory. There may be gaps of time missing from his memory. It's going to take until 4:00 p.m. on Friday for his BAC to come back down to zero. And one last big bummer: when he first woke up, he was greeted with the inevitable price that must be paid for excessive drinking—the hangover.

## Hangovers

Oh, my dear God, *make it stop*! Headache. Dry mouth. Dizzy. Nauseous. Exhausted. Yup, you're hungover. There are plenty of myths about how to free yourself from the hellish prison you're stuck in, but only one thing will altogether remove the negative side effects: time.[27] As we discussed earlier, your liver can only process alcohol so fast, so when you stockpiled all those drinks last night (Connor, you animal), you gave your body the task of returning to "normal." Depending on how much you had, it could take hours—maybe even most of the next day. You may have friends with brilliant ideas about how to feel better, like "hair of the dog" (having another alcoholic drink in the morning) or eating greasy food. Neither of those will help beyond instant gratification, and both will, ultimately, make you feel worse. However, here are five things you *can* do to ease the suffering:

1. **Drink Water.** It might not sound sexy, but drinking water will help you rebalance your hydration levels and alleviate some of the awfulness you are experiencing. It's going to take most of the day to get your hydration back on track, so continue to push water. It may not seem appetizing—get over it. Although alcoholic drinks are predominantly made up of water (beer is 95 percent water), it doesn't matter. Alcohol is a diuretic, meaning it causes you to pee more than you usually would. When you consume booze, you will always end up with a net loss of water from your system.[28] So drink up! Water, I mean.

2. **Pump Up Those Electrolytes.** All the peeing is going to lead to a loss of minerals such as sodium, potassium, and magnesium, which are crucial to muscle function, mental focus, and body cooling.[29] To correct the imbalance, eat potassium-rich foods like bananas and spinach, have a glass of coconut water, or take a trip to your local drugstore for a bottle of Pedialyte, which contains twice as much sodium and five times as much potassium as Gatorade (not to mention, a fraction of the sugar). Pedialyte was created to help rehydrate vomiting, diarrhea-ridden toddlers, which is exactly what a nasty hangover will turn you into. It doesn't taste great, but it's effective and will help you feel better.

3. **Eat.** You need to eat. It doesn't have to be a full meal, but you should eat something. You may be craving greasy comfort foods, but try to avoid them, as they can further irritate your stomach. Sugary foods may seem like a great idea—*God, I just want to feel happy*—but the inevitable crash that follows will likely add to your depressive deficit. I would tell you to order some prickly pear cactus extract, as some research suggests it can help fight hangovers,[30] but come on, is that really something you're going to do? Instead, grab some food like eggs or yogurt, which are loaded with amino acids like cysteine that help boost liver function, or oatmeal, which can help restore magnesium and balance acids in your body.[31] Fruit and fruit juices have been shown to reduce suffering; just be careful with how much sugar you're pumping into your decrepit vessel of a body.[32]

4. **Take Ibuprofen.** I'm sure your head is pounding, but stay away from over-the-counter pain relievers that contain acetaminophen (like Tylenol). The combination with alcohol can be even more taxing on the liver.[33] Instead, reach for products with the active ingredient ibuprofen (Advil, Motrin). They can help reduce your headache without putting your liver through any more stress.

5. **Exercise?** If you smell like booze the morning after drinking, there's a simple explanation—alcohol is still in your system. Alcohol is a toxin, and when you drink too much of it, you became intoxicated. Pretty gross, right? Some people may suggest getting some exercise to sweat out the toxins. While there is *some* truth to the concept, the amount is minuscule—about 90 percent of the alcohol you consume will be processed by your liver,[34] not sweat out through your pores. If working out is something you're up for, more power to you. Exercising will release some feel-good endorphins. But remember that you are already dehydrated. Any additional water loss from sweat could further exacerbate dehydration symptoms and will require you to consume even more water to get back to normal hydration levels.

## Heavy Stuff

Things are about to get a little dark, but have no fear! I promise we won't dwell on anything too long. This stuff can get a bit heavy, but it's important, worth knowing, and, frankly, really crazy.

### Greek Life

Frats and sororities are not inherently scary or dangerous. You are not a bad person or a mindless sheep for joining; it may actually provide some of the most memorable experiences of your life that could be overwhelmingly positive. However, what does deserve a close examination is the relationship between fraternities, sororities, and alcohol.

*"Greek life has such a presence on a lot of college campuses throughout the country and, at least here, most fraternities are centered around drinking a lot."*

—UNIVERSITY OF RICHMOND, SOPHOMORE

The pros of joining a fraternity or sorority are understandably enticing. A frequently touted perk is the network of alumni professionals that can help with careers postgraduation. Some houses even have private chefs that make your meals. *Denver omelet with cheddar, please!* However, the most immediate benefit of Greek life is that it gives new students instant access to friends and community. An entire social sphere. It's scary and lonely to be in a new place without friends, and joining these groups provides social comfort and structure, not to mention parties. Fraternities and sororities throw a number of parties throughout each semester that are only meant for members and/or recruits.

*"Joining Greek life automatically gave me a key to all public and private parties on and off campus, as well as events between houses. There are parties at least four nights out of the week with endless drinks, music, and fun people. I would say I definitely started drinking more because I joined Greek life."*
—UNIVERSITY OF CALIFORNIA, LOS ANGELES, FRESHMAN

As much fun as Greek life can be, however, the downsides are numerous and dire, beginning with hazing. At least one student has died every single year since 1969 in a hazing ritual, nearly all connected with a fraternity or sorority.[35] Most deaths are due to alcohol poisoning or some irreparable physical harm suffered while intoxicated, like falling down stairs, falling off a bridge, or being punched repeatedly in the kidneys.

In 2017, a junior at Florida State University was found unresponsive the morning after a frat party. It was discovered that he had been coerced into drinking an entire bottle of bourbon and died of alcohol poisoning in the hours after. The coroner estimated his blood alcohol content at the time of death was .55. He was twenty years old. Earlier in the same semester, a freshman at LSU was pledging and died of acute alcohol intoxication and aspiration (he stopped breathing) after consuming the equivalent of twenty-four shots.[36] His BAC at his time of death was .49. He was in the third week of his freshman year. He was eighteen years old.

Fraternities and sororities circumstantially place enormous pressure on freshmen to participate in heavy binge drinking. Sorority members are nearly twice as likely to be binge drinkers compared to nonsorority female students (62 percent versus 35 percent, respectively). Among women who live in sorority houses, an astonishing 80 percent binge drink.[37] Similarly, fraternity members binge more than other male students (75 percent versus 45 percent, respectively), and 86 percent of fraternity house residents binge drink.[38]

*"As a member of Greek life I will go out and drink heavily at least three times a week. This includes pregaming with my closest friends, then once we get to the party, we'll drink a considerable amount more."*

—INDIANA UNIVERSITY, FRESHMAN

While this behavior may seem isolated to the *time* of being in college and the *conditions* of living in fraternity/sorority houses, many people continue binge drinking well into adulthood. A longitudinal study of nearly twenty thousand individuals found that close to half of fraternity members report symptoms of alcohol use disorder by the age of thirty-five.[39] *Close to HALF!* It's pretty incredible to be able to segment a part of the population by two factors (male, participated in Greek life), and be able to predict that *almost half* of them, statistically speaking, will have a drinking problem.

Don't get me wrong. There are great sororities and fraternities that do amazing outreach, don't haze their pledges to tears, and kick out (rather than idolize) members who make dangerous and stupid decisions while drinking. The goal is to surround yourself with people who make good choices and want the best for you, and if you can find that group in a sorority or fraternity, then that's where you should be. Just know there are risks associated with being a part of that world, so choose both the houses you pledge and the one you join carefully if you end up going that route.

## Angry Drunks

College nightlife spots are frequently filled with people who are wasted. The larger the crowd, the higher the chance that you will be near someone who overdid it. It's important to understand what drunk people look and act like, so you can avoid those that are beyond the point of reason and could be harmful. *That guy just knocked down a stop sign, and now he's wearing it like a necklace and . . . wait, no, he threw it. He threw the stop sign like a Frisbee. And he's picking it up again. Let's go the other way.*

Almost 700,000 students a year are physically assaulted by another student under the influence of alcohol.[40] Let that marinate for a minute. That's the population of Baltimore or Milwaukee, and significantly more than Kansas City, Atlanta, or Miami. And that's *every* year! When overconsumed, alcohol affects the brain's ability to assess risk. It dampens how you perceive sights and sounds and impairs physical control. And when your BAC rises into the range above .125, it can make you angry.

The Harvard CAS also discovered that "students who attended schools with high rates of binge drinking experienced a greater number of secondhand effects, including disruption of sleep or study, property damage; and verbal, physical, or sexual violence, than their peers attending schools with low binge drinking rates."[41]

*"In a crowded bar, I accidentally nudged someone. I apologized, but the guy hit me anyway. He struck me in the face with a pitcher, dousing me with beer and making my mouth bleed."*
—COLLEGE ALCOHOL STUDY[42]

Whether you're at a fraternity party or a college bar, your proximity to drunk people, especially as the night gets later and later, puts you in a potentially dangerous situation. Stay aware of your surroundings, leave when things get crazy, and make sure you're in the company of people you trust.

*"Do not drink when you are sad, tired, or angry. It will only make you more sad, tired, or angry. It may seem like alcohol will take away hard feelings, but it doesn't work that way."*
—GEORGETOWN UNIVERSITY, SOPHOMORE

## Sexual Assault

> **Trigger Warning:** The next section may be difficult to read. It involves accounts of sexual assault, consent, and alcohol that may cue intense emotional responses. Please proceed only if you feel comfortable.

Sexual assault is disgustingly common in college. My mother was assaulted during her freshman year, and unfortunately, this type of behavior still occurs with startling frequency. About one hundred thousand students report alcohol-related sexual assaults every year,[43] though the actual figure is much higher, as more than 90 percent of victims on campuses choose not to report their assaults.[44] A study from 2016 shows one in five female students will experience a sexual assault while in college.[45] *One in five.* Think of five women you know. No, really. Think of five. Why does this happen? Well, the answer is complicated. There's lots of research currently being done about how we, as a society, raise boys into young men—how they view sex, consent, and respect. How they deal with anger, rejection, and embarrassment. There's also plenty to be said about the prevalence and availability of hard-core pornography that, frequently, reduces women to pleasure objects for male entertainment. However, the presence of one particular factor increases the likelihood of sexual violence: alcohol.

*"I've heard stories about people running away during parties because of how drunk they were. Unfortunately, a close friend of mine was raped at a party. I haven't been through too much as a result of drinking, but I know people who have. I've been fortunate."*

—UNIVERSITY OF CALIFORNIA, LOS ANGELES, FRESHMAN

We're not suggesting alcohol is solely responsible for criminal behavior. Still, the link between overconsumption of alcohol and sexual assault is undeniable. It is estimated that 50 percent of rapes are committed by someone who is under the influence,[46] and up to 72 percent occur while the victim is intoxicated.[47] Sexual assault on college campuses is most likely to occur at the beginning of the school year, on either a Friday or Saturday, between the hours of midnight and 6:00 a.m.[48] Essentially, the most obvious times for parties.

It probably will not surprise you that the vast majority of these crimes—more than 90 percent—are committed by men.[49] Gentlemen—we have to do better. This isn't just about making sure *you're* never responsible for sexual violence, it's about making a moral choice to help protect people. That means noticing when someone is drunk and understanding what they may be capable of *because* they're drunk. Whether it's a friend who's aggressively pursuing someone or a friend who might appear drunk and "out of it," it's our personal and social obligation to stop this type of behavior if we see it. The unfortunate truth is that this problem starts with men, and we have to be a part of a solution. I'm not trying to oversimplify the social pressures of being a young man, and I'm not suggesting that you're now expected to be some superhero. What I think you should strive for—what, hopefully, all of us can strive for—is being a good person. Because of the prevalence of partying and people pushing their limits, college is unfortunately plagued with sexual assault, and you have the opportunity to make a difference at your school. As I mentioned before, plenty of researchers are trying to figure out not only why this happens, but what to do to make tangible changes in the behavior of young men. A common theme is respect for and an understanding of consent.

*"I went to a fraternity party off campus. I had at least twelve shots of liquor and two mixed drinks. That night I went home with this guy that I did not know and had sex with him. The guy and his roommates carried me home to my dorm, where two RAs caught me. I went to the hospital for alcohol poisoning and rape. I blacked out. I never pressed charges because he used the condom in my wallet."*
—COLLEGE ALCOHOL STUDY[50]

For many students, the college experience includes sex, and I cannot stress enough the importance of being on the same page as your partner. According to one large university's website, "affirmative consent is when someone agrees, gives permission, or says 'yes' to sexual activity with other persons. It is always freely given, and all people in a sexual situation must feel that they are able to say 'yes' or 'no' or stop the sexual activity at any point."[51] Consent is yours and yours alone to give, and cannot be coerced or demanded. When either person has been drinking, things can quickly become legally and morally complicated, especially if someone is drunk. When alcohol is consumed excessively, its handicapping effects can be so strong that a person may not be able to give consent. If someone is too intoxicated to communicate clearly, they are too intoxicated to give consent. Just in case anyone wasn't listening. IF SOMEONE IS TOO INTOXICATED TO COMMUNICATE, THEY ARE TOO INTOXICATED TO GIVE CONSENT. Let's unpack this for a second because it's really frickin' important.

It is always the responsibility of the person who initiates sexual contact to obtain consent. I know that sounds pretty clinical, but if you're putting on the moves, it is *your* legal obligation to find out if your advances are welcomed. In case it's not perfectly clear, if a person is too drunk to communicate that they want to have sex, stop. Having sex with someone who is too drunk to give consent is a form of sexual assault called incapacitated rape. It's a crime. *Remember Brock Turner?* He was sentenced to six months in jail and must register as a sex offender for life. And the young woman he assaulted? You should read her incredibly powerful statement she gave during his sentencing. Frankly, it should be required reading for every freshman. Unless you've experienced a sexual assault, I'm not sure it's possible to truly fathom the damage it causes. What we can do is listen, try our best to understand, and be aware of the situations that facilitate these tragedies. A 2015 study conducted by researchers from Brown University and Syracuse University found that 15 percent of college freshmen surveyed had experienced an incapacitated rape.[52] *That's only freshmen!*

If you ever find yourself in a sexual situation that is uncomfortable or does not feel safe, stopping is always an option. Even if you initially wanted to go down that road, and then changed your mind, you can always say, "I want to stop." I completely recognize that, as a man, this may be easy for me to say. The abundance of social pressures placed on women is something I will never experience, nor could I ever claim to understand how difficult it would be to stop someone's unwanted sexual advances—especially someone larger who could make me fear for my safety. I hope you are never put in such a terrible situation. It is gut-wrenching how often these events take place, but the pervasiveness of sexual misconduct on college campuses is a reality that every incoming freshman should be warned about. It pains me to write these words, but you need to know what to do if this happens to you.

Someone we know and love was sexually assaulted on a major college campus while we were working on this project. She had been drinking and enlisted the help of a sober friend to walk her home. He stuck around after they arrived, and then he assaulted her. She was drunk. He was sober. This was someone she knew. Someone she trusted. Someone she would inevitably see again.

The multitude of factors leading to our society being anything but appalled at sexual assault deserves examination beyond what we can supply in this book, but we can at least provide a starting point for an action plan. Stories from survivors are incredibly important for our entire population in order to better educate society at large about this epidemic. Although rehashing the past was difficult, our loved one generously offered to share her experience in hopes that it would help others feel less alone.

*"The morning after I was assaulted, I wasn't sure what to do. Who could I confide in? What would I say? Would they blame me for what happened? My mind was filled with second guesses and doubts. The one thing that stood out to me was what every activist, orientation program, and risk workshop had stressed: speak up.*

*Luckily, I had a friend working for my university's police department and asked him to accompany me to file a report so I wouldn't be alone. He didn't ask me any questions, which made me feel like he didn't judge me, pressure me to talk about it, and wasn't interested in talking to anyone else about my situation. Find a friend who respects your privacy. File a report as soon as possible, while your memory is fresh. It does not need to be followed up with an investigation; you can just ask to have the incident on record.*

*Months later, I'm glad I filed a report so soon since my memories are fading, and I'm trying to forget what happened. However, what was more difficult for me was approaching my parents. I felt comfortable talking to a few of my closest friends, knowing they would be a solid support system. I thought that unlike my friends, my parents would be upset with me or push it under the rug. I didn't want to add negativity to their lives, have them see their daughter in a different light, or blame themselves or their parenting for what happened.*

*Two months after the incident, I finally got the courage to sit down with them. They responded with more support and love than I could have imagined. Their number one priority since our discussion has been me and my needs, and they immediately started to ask around their circles for someone who could recommend a therapist, legal counseling, and Title IX expertise. I'd like to hope that most parents respond this way. Even if you're unsure about coming forward to your parent(s), you might be surprised at what resources and experiences they can share to make sure you heal.*

*The final piece that started me on my path to recovery was reaching out to campus resources such as the Title IX and Campus Assault Resources and Education Offices. All colleges and universities receiving any kind of federal funding (public or private—likely most campuses) are mandated to have Title IX resources on campus. Find yours and reach out. These counselors and experts have received specialized training to handle all varieties of sexual assault, and they are the best people to help you find your custom path to recovery since not everyone's is the same.*

*As a survivor of sexual assault, I cannot stress enough how important it is to speak up and reach out. There are entire offices on campus designed to help you, and your friends and family may have a few tricks up their sleeve to get you the resources you need. I cannot imagine my recovery process if I hadn't gotten some kind of guidance, and I know that it helped me realize that I am still empowered, especially as a survivor."*

**What to Do If You've Been Sexually Assaulted.** If you are sexually assaulted, *it is not your fault*, no matter the circumstances. Should you ever need it, here is a list of what to do if you've been sexually assaulted.[53]

- **Call 911** if you're in immediate danger, otherwise . . .
- **Get to a safe place.**
- **If you were assaulted by a stranger, write down everything you can remember.** Details about the person and what happened will be helpful in making a clear statement to police and medical professionals.
- **Talk to someone about reporting the assault.** You can call the National Sexual Assault Hotline (800-656-HOPE) to talk to a trained professional about how to report the crime.
- **If the person who harmed you is a fellow student, report it to school authorities.** The school has an obligation to help you continue your education and will take the necessary means to make sure contact between you and the perpetrator is limited.
- **Reach out for help.** The staff at a hospital, campus medical center, or campus counseling center will be able to point you in the direction of counseling that could be helpful after a sexual assault. Give yourself time to heal. There are resources on your campus to help you cope with what's happened.

If you've been raped (a form of sexual assault that specifically refers to penetration without consent):

- **Don't wash or clean your body.** The physical evidence on your body can be important for police, so do your best to resist changing your clothes, showering, brushing your teeth, or combing your hair. As quickly as possible . . .
- **Get medical care.** Call 911 or go to your nearest hospital emergency room. Tell them that you've been sexually assaulted and that you need help. You will likely receive medicine to prevent STDs and emergency contraception to prevent pregnancy, then a doctor or nurse will use a rape kit to collect evidence. **You do not need to press charges in order to have evidence collected with a rape kit, and you do not need to decide to press charges while at the hospital.**

Between 80 and 90 percent of sexual assaults involve two people who know each other.[54] The perpetrator may not even know they have violated consent or some other boundary until after the fact, which is why it is so explicitly important to clearly establish whether or not consent has been given before anything happens.

It seems inappropriate for me to tell you that you *have to* report the incident if you're sexually assaulted, as I feel unqualified to assume the role of understanding the scope of complications involved and enormous strength required to take action. What I can tell you is that you have rights and that you are not alone. If you are having trouble finding who to call and where to go, start with your student health center, campus police/safety enforcement, and the local police near your school. It won't be easy speaking to strangers about your experience, and finding the words to communicate what happened to you may be painful. Start with your name. Tell them you've been sexually assaulted and that you need help.

As mentioned in the passage earlier, you *and* your body are protected by law in this country. In 1972, Congress passed crucial legislation into law called Title IX. It guarantees legal protections against sexual harassment and sexual assault for students in schools that receive federal funding. Since pretty much all schools receive funding in the form of federal financial aid, this should be available at whatever college or university you attend. After filing an internal complaint with your school, they are required to do what they can to prevent further harassment or violence, which might include "changing your class schedule, prohibiting the perpetrator from contacting you, or even taking disciplinary action against the perpetrator."[55]

If you have more questions about Title IX protections or want to know what to do if you feel your school isn't handling complaints properly, the website for the American Association of University Women (aauw.org) is an excellent resource. If you aren't ready to talk to anyone yet, but want step-by-step guidance about how to proceed after a sexual assault, the website for the Office on Women's Health (womenshealth.gov) is an excellent place to start.

## Alcohol Use Disorder

Almost done with all the heavy talk! Drinking booze helps tons of people have a good time and do so responsibly. Frankly, the vast majority of college students

(80 percent) do not meet the criteria for "having a drinking problem."[56] It's comforting to know that most people who drink have a healthy relationship with alcohol, but I don't happen to be one of them. I stopped drinking because I, frankly, couldn't handle it. I regularly drank too much, and even though I'd go long stretches of drinking responsibly, the bad habits I developed were too easy to eventually fall back into. For me, all of these patterns were solidified in college. And while the majority of my peers didn't share my drinking problems, I certainly wasn't alone. The other 20 percent of college students meet the criteria for suffering from alcohol use disorder, so if you're wondering, *Hmm . . . could this be me?*, the yes/no questions below can help provide some clarity.[57]

The following eleven criteria for alcohol use disorder are outlined in the fifth edition of the *Diagnostic and Statistical Manual of Mental Disorders* (*DSM-5*).[58] The number of positive responses is used to judge severity, with a score of two to three for a mild disorder, four to five for moderate, and six and above for severe. Here are the questions, as listed by the National Institute on Alcohol Abuse and Alcoholism:

In the past year, have you:

- More than once wanted to cut down or stop drinking, or tried to, but couldn't?
- Spent a lot of time drinking? Or being sick or getting over the aftereffects?
- Experienced craving—a strong need, or urge, to drink?
- Found that drinking—or being sick from drinking—often interfered with taking care of your home or family? Or caused job troubles? Or school problems?
- Continued to drink even though it was causing trouble with your family or friends?
- Given up or cut back on activities that were important or interesting to you, or gave you pleasure, in order to drink?
- More than once gotten into situations while or after drinking that increased your chances of getting hurt (such as driving, swimming, using machinery, walking in a dangerous area, or having unsafe sex)?
- Continued to drink even though it was making you feel depressed or anxious or adding to another health problem? Or after having had a memory blackout?

- Had to drink much more than you once did to get the effect you want? Or found that your usual number of drinks had much less effect than before?
- Found that when the effects of alcohol were wearing off, you had withdrawal symptoms, such as trouble sleeping, shakiness, irritability, anxiety, depression, restlessness, nausea, or sweating? Or sensed things that were not there?

I knew I had a problem long before I asked for help. If you can be there for a person who needs this type of help, it is truly one of the greatest gifts you can give. If you feel like you may have a problem with alcohol, I can promise you that you are not alone. The best thing you can do is talk to a medical professional. Verbalizing your struggles and gathering professional feedback can help you begin the process of evaluating the role that alcohol plays in your life and how to best move forward.

---

If someone you know is suffering from alcohol abuse disorder, your ability to help them is completely contingent on their motivation to help themselves. You cannot force someone to seek help. First off, it'll never work if they're not interested, but it's also the law. Only extreme circumstances, such as a violent incident resulting in court-ordered treatment or a medical emergency, can force a person to seek help. If they are unwilling, you must not make it your burden. What you can do is talk to them, and more importantly, listen. The following are talking points recommended by professionals that can help you be there for someone who may need it:[59]

- **Discuss recent incidents.** Talk to your friend shortly after a night gone badly, but choose a time when you're both sober, calm, and have a private place to chat.
- **Use examples.** Be clear with your friend that you care about them, and you're worried about their drinking, then give specific instances where you've seen their consumption of booze cause a problem.
- **Get help.** Gather information in advance about treatment options on your campus. If the person is willing to receive guidance, offer to go with them to their first visit with a counselor.

## Be Smart

We're done! That was sobering, right? *Get it?* Are we having fun yet? Listen, it is absolutely possible to enjoy alcohol in college, drink responsibly, and avoid the dangerous pitfalls that accompany overindulgence. If you decide *this* is what you want to do, you *can* do it. All too often, ignorance is to blame for people making terrible decisions associated with alcohol. But now you know things. Like your limit. And the fact that you shouldn't chug liquor. Or accept a drink someone else made for you for a variety of reasons. Try not to take shots. Don't ever drive when you've been drinking, and don't ride with people who've been drinking. Okay, okay—I'll stop soapboxing. I'm sure some (if not all) of this has been a little overwhelming, but you can do this. In fact, because you are now on your own, *only* you can do this.

## For When You Forget

Because booze can be fun and make us feel good . . . until it doesn't. When you're ready to take control of your relationship with alcohol, start here:

- **Quantity *and* Time Matter.** Keep track of not only *how much* you are drinking, but also *how often*. Consuming alcohol too quickly will result in a sudden spike in your BAC, overwhelming your liver's ability to process it and setting you up for a slew of negative side effects. To help manage consumption over time, drink water in between drinks.
- **Find Your Ceiling.** This is the number of drinks that you should never surpass, ever, something like, "I *never* drink more than three drinks." Use your weight, sex, and a BAC chart to get a baseline understanding of how many drinks will raise your BAC to .12 over the course of a few hours. Don't go past this number in a night. What lies beyond is nothing but bad stuff: blackouts, vomiting, stupor, coma, death . . . bad. Remember, people die every year from drinking. If you've hit your ceiling and someone tries to get you to drink more, repeat the words, "No thanks, I'm good," over and over until they leave you alone.
- **Set Your Limit for the Night.** This doesn't have to be the same as your ceiling. Having a plan for how much you want to drink will help you stay on

track when euphoria kicks in. This doesn't mean that you can't ever change your mind or adjust on the fly, but being conscious and deliberate about how many drinks you plan on having will help keep you from making mistakes.

Try to remember:

- **Go Out with People Who Have Your Back.** Befriend those who also want to drink responsibly. Stay together and look out for one another. Bad things can happen around really drunk people. Be able to identify when someone is intoxicated and be aware of their proximity to you. Also, know the signs and symptoms of the later stages of intoxication, and don't be afraid to call for help if you're worried about a friend. Why? Because . . .

- **Alcohol Is Poison.** Drinking a lot of poison really fast is a terrible idea. You could die. Your safety is your responsibility now. Have fun, be safe, and most importantly, take care of yourself out there. You've got this.

# CHAPTER 4

# EXERCISE

$$\boxed{\text{JILL}}$$

**Despite having coached high school sports for nearly fifteen years, I'm not a natural athlete.** Particularly in my early years, I was objectively terrible on every sports team I was a part of. In third grade, I used to whisper to my softball mitt, "Please, for the love of God, catch the ball." The mitt didn't listen. When I was benched during middle school basketball because I couldn't dribble, my dad put a Nerf hoop in our living room to boost my confidence. Seven days after the install, I caved in the three vertical feet of the Sheetrock wall that was holding the hoop while attempting a layup. That's right. I completely destroyed *an interior wall* with just my hip and shoulder. My dad wasn't even mad, which still amazes me—in his words, "Shit happens when you go hard"—though he did write "JILL WAS HERE" in giant Sharpie letters on the wall with an arrow pointing to the damage in case clarity was required. He thought this was hilarious. I laughed at first, stopping only when I realized that his homemade graffiti was going to have to stay up until he repaired the wall, which didn't happen for six months. Precisely the confidence builder that every thirteen-year-old needs.

Long runs during track practice in high school gave me an excuse to visit the local candy shop. Unfortunately, jelly beans didn't improve my two-hundred-meter time. Still, I *was* honored with an award at the end of my senior year, the "Biggest

Nut," which was apparently given to the most enthusiastic participant. I may not have been fast, but I happened to have a real gift for speech giving—a talent that I also shared with those on my soccer team. Though I wasn't good at that sport either, I played a particularly important role as a senior: delivering the pump-up speech before every game. In the interest of originality, one of my teammates and I created one that involved milking an imaginary cow while screaming, "*Udder* Domination!" It killed every time. Though I always loved the games, saying goodbye to practice when I graduated high school was a relief. Little did I know I was saying goodbye to the only reason I was exercising.

Exercise in high school is easy if you play a sport. All you have to do is make the decision to join a team, and the rest is done for you. You're told when to show up and what to do, and you have coaches and teammates to show you how to do it. When all of that ends after high school, exercise is a different beast. Suddenly you're accountable to no one other than yourself. You have to set aside time, make a plan, show up, and, to work hard, you have to push *yourself*. All of that makes sticking with it much more challenging. Every year I'm personally reminded of just how brutal the transition from high school sports to working out on your own is. From June to December, I train with my cross-country team and get to experience the same benefits of the structure and accountability that my athletes do. Exercising is effortless during that period. It's built into my life. The end of the season is always sobering. I miss the team and coaching, but the biggest transition is being totally on my own again with exercise.

*"Throughout my childhood and even through high school, I was almost always on a sports team, so the majority of my exercise came from organized sports. I never learned to exercise on my own; I didn't know what to do in a gym, and I wasn't used to dragging myself out for a run if I didn't have a coach or teammates relying on me to show up. It took me a long time to learn to exercise independently (and to be honest, I still haven't totally figured it out)."*
—STANFORD UNIVERSITY, RECENT GRAD

Being a three-sport athlete in high school seemed to make exercising alone even harder for me once I got to college. During the break between seasons in high school, I never exercised. I'd come home, put on sweatpants, watch something stupid while eating an absurdly large bowl of ice cream, and then nap until just before my parents got home. I went into full sloth mode. My parents, though unimpressed, never got on my case because it was only a week or two. Unfortunately, it was easy to fall into that same familiar pattern during my freshman year of college, when afternoon practice ceased to exist because sports were completely gone from my life. I had never figured out how to exercise on my own, and more importantly, *I didn't care to try.* The only effort I was regularly exerting in the afternoon was walking from the fridge to the couch and back. Furthermore, there was seemingly no consequence of spending time that way.

My story is a common one for high school athletes. Once exercise becomes optional, it's easy to opt out. The novelty of being lazy is incredibly appealing, at least at first. But when the charm wears off, and that type of behavior starts to make your body feel gross, you'll finally come to realize that you don't know how to turn that train around. So, you'll either half-ass an exercise routine or ignore the necessity of movement altogether because you don't think you can make it stick. At least that's what I did, vacillating between those two outcomes for two years before figuring out how to incorporate exercise in a way that would last.

*"In high school, it was easy for me to exercise and not think about it because I was always in a sport, even in summer. In college, I completely stopped. I was totally unmotivated."*

—COLLEGE OF WILLIAM AND MARY, JUNIOR

If you weren't an athlete in high school or you stopped playing sports midway through, then you've already considered the role exercise plays in your life. There are three ways this shakes out for most people: (a) you know exercise is important, and whether you enjoy it or not, you've found a way to hold yourself accountable and have established a regular workout routine; (b) you know you should exercise more and feel bad that you don't, but you've got other stuff going on and don't have time to make it a standard part of your week; (c) you don't like exercise, don't do it, and don't feel bad about it.

It's hard to get the (a), and it doesn't happen by chance for most people. If you're not there yet, you're in the vast majority. Nearly 75 percent of American adults state that they *want* to be in shape. Still, only 30 percent consider exercise to be one of their habits,[1] and only 23 percent meet the US Department of Health and Human Services exercise recommendation of 150 minutes of cardio and two sessions of strength each week.[2,3] For many people, exercise is just plain hard—physically and mentally—and frankly, excuses are easier to make than commitments.

*"When it comes to exercise, there is always something better to do. There is always somebody to hang out with, or homework to do, or a chore that is more important."*

—INDIANA UNIVERSITY, FRESHMAN

Getting started is particularly difficult. Studies have shown that 50 percent of people who begin an exercise routine give up within six months.[4] It takes planning and regular effort to add exercise to your life in a sustainable way, but I promise if you do it, you'll be so grateful for the role it plays. It wasn't easy for me to replace ice cream and long naps with a daily workout. To get there, I had to mindfully establish some specifics: *why* I wanted to exercise, *when* I was going to do it, and *what* I was going to do.

We're not big believers in the quick fix, particularly when it comes to exercise. We all start at different levels of fitness, come at it with varying degrees of enthusiasm, and are intimidated by different things. There's no one way to involve movement in your life, and there's certainly no one way that works for everyone. There are, however, a few universal considerations that are required to make it stick, whatever your goals. The first is that you need to have a reason to get after it, so we're going to talk about some of the physical and mental benefits of exercise in hopes that one of them will pique your interest. That's where you're going to establish your *why*. Next, we'll discuss timing, because exercise unfortunately only happens if you actively set aside time for it and show up, which I've always found to be the hardest part. We'll end the chapter with a rundown of the many ways you can exercise, giving some specific workout routine ideas in places where it makes sense. I'll cite a fair deal of research in this chapter, but I'm also going to talk a lot about what has worked for me and what I've seen work for others when it comes to exercise.

The ultimate goal is that you end this chapter with a metaphorical fishing rod. More directly, we want you to be able to confidently craft your own workout plan so that you never need to be told how to exercise again but rather have the knowledge of what to do and can create the necessary accountability to follow through. So, saddle up, it's go time!

## Why Bother

For anything that requires a decent amount of your time and energy, you should force yourself to answer the question, "Why?" This goes for jobs, side projects, favors, outings, and relationships as much as it goes for working out. As far as exercise is concerned, your *why* can change as you go, but it's essential that you always have one. When excuses start to sound appealing, that very *why* will help you deflect them. It'll keep you grounded in your reason for beginning a routine in the first place. According to one sizeable study on a university campus, the best predictor of exercise frequency and duration for both men and women is holding the belief that working out is important for your identity, consistent with your personal values, and will result in outcomes that are of value to you.[5] Bottom line—you'll need a *why* to make exercise a regular habit. Here are six *whys* worth considering.

1. **You Want to Look Good Naked.** Gaining or sustaining body confidence is the reason most people start to work out. It's certainly what got me going. A national study found that more than 80 percent of people exercise because they want to feel good about their body.[6] It's hard not to be motivated by the promise of bright skin, toned muscles, and decreased body fat that comes from working out. Stick with exercise, and you might be contacting the art department to see if they need any nude models before too long.

> *"What drives me to go to the gym five or six times a week, even when I just want to stay in bed and watch Netflix, is that I want to look good. I feel more confident when I work out—I carry myself differently. I feel more comfortable in my body. Especially in an environment as socially oriented as college is, anything to make yourself more comfortable is a plus."*
> —NORTHWESTERN UNIVERSITY, JUNIOR

2. **You Want to Be in Top Physical and Mental Shape.** Once I got in shape and gained confidence in my body, this became my *why*. It still is. When you know what it's like to feel good as a result of exercise, you'll start to crave it, which is great because it's a wonder drug for lifelong health. Studies have shown that it's the safest way to prevent *and* treat many chronic illnesses and physical ailments.[7] It's also proven to combat some of the biggest mental health challenges you may face while in college: stress, anxiety, depression, and low energy levels, to name a few. Additionally, it strengthens your immune system, which you'll be grateful for when that annual plague hits campus.[8]

> *"Lack of incentive makes it easy to never exercise, but I need to for my mental health. It's how I manage stress."*
>
> —OBERLIN COLLEGE, SENIOR

Getting moderate exercise has been found to increase life span by more than twelve years when combined with healthy eating and reduced smoking and drinking.[9] Physical activity alone has also been found to decrease the risk of heart disease by up to 41 percent,[10] as well as improve circulation, prevent bone loss, and reduce the risk of certain cancers.[11] While you probably don't spend much time thinking about getting older, your future self will thank you for doing anything that buys you more time. Aging seems to suck supremely, but it will take much less of a toll on your body if you're healthy. To take advantage of those benefits, however, you've got to get started. Research suggests that it becomes tough to establish new habits after the age of thirty.[12] Thus, incorporating an exercise routine when you're young increases the odds that you'll continue moving throughout your life.

3. **You Love Setting Goals and Working Toward Them.** What's more satisfying than seeing improvement? With a goal in mind, you'll view exercise as training, which will make it easier for you to show up and stay focused. The key when setting goals is to make them SMART: specific, measurable, achievable, relevant, and time-based. Instead of planning to just "get stronger," set a more specific intention, like bench pressing a particular weight by the end of the semester. Rather than a general "get faster," shoot for running a 5K under a specific time. I break my yearly exercise calendar down by season and set fitness

goals during the fall and spring. During those periods, my focus is on getting faster or stronger, while during the winter and summer, I exercise to maintain my baseline. This approach works well with a school schedule because you can set one goal per semester, but you might also con-

*"It's addicting to see improvements in my speed and gains in my strength. Those changes motivate me to stick with my workouts."*

—PITZER COLLEGE, FRESHMAN

sider switching it, setting goals during periods that you're on break and have more time to exercise. However, I typically find that having a goal when I am busy is precisely what I need to stick to my routine. When I'm working toward an objective, I'm more likely to fit exercise into my crammed schedule.

4. **You Need Some Time Alone.** Use exercise to quiet the world when you need to be alone. You will constantly be surrounded by others—your roommate, people on your floor, people in your classes, and people in your clubs—it will feel relentless at some point. *I love you all, but if you don't leave, I'm going to explode.* Take time for yourself during your workouts. Listen to a podcast, stream a show, listen to the music you're too embarrassed to play without headphones on. Spending time alone can be exactly what you need to refocus and recharge.

*"I love that I get to listen to music and not be accountable to texts/emails coming in for an hour of my day. Exercise can be social, but I love that it is my time, just me and my thoughts and my music and my body getting stronger."*

—GEORGETOWN UNIVERSITY, SOPHOMORE

5. **You're Craving Balance.** To maintain total body health, you'll need to achieve balance with several major areas in college, such as schoolwork, eating, and partying. Exercise can be the perfect positive behavior to put on the other side of the seesaw.

Taking a break from studying to exercise will positively contribute to the quality of your work, as physical activity improves memory recall and storage, helps with impulse control, and sharpens focus for several hours afterward, all resulting in greater productivity.[13] So, instead of pressing pause midpaper to eat a whole pizza or take a power nap, try going for a short run or fast walk. Countless articles and books have been written about the secrets of highly successful people, and perhaps unsurprisingly, exercise is a foundational part of the day for nearly all of those who kick ass for a living.[14]

*"You're either going to drink a lot in college or eat terrible food (or both). Your body won't be able to keep up unless you exercise."*

—FORDHAM UNIVERSITY, JUNIOR

As far as the environment is concerned, exercise will be essential to your health if you're not interested in setting boundaries where food and booze are concerned. There's a saying that you "can't outrun your fork," but exercise will undoubtedly push you closer to breaking even as far as calories in versus out.

6. **You Want to See Your Friends.** Exercising while catching up with a friend kills two birds with one stone. Plus, it's cheaper than eating out, healthier than drinking, and more productive than binge-watching shows together on a computer. What's more, friends provide accountability, as they replace the teammates you might have had in high school. It's easier to show up when you know you'll be letting someone else down if you don't.

*"I see exercise as an excuse to relieve stress and hang out with my friends. That way, we can be stressed together and catch up while also being productive in a nonacademic way."*
—GEORGE WASHINGTON UNIVERSITY, SENIOR

7. **You Want to Make New Friends.** Joining a team or going to a fitness class can also be a great way to meet new people. The endorphins released through exercise can boost happiness and make you feel carefree—the perfect state of mind for putting yourself out there. And speaking of putting yourself out there, if you're looking for romance, exercise might also be the ticket. Not just because you'll look better naked, but because exercise induces the same physiological symptoms as arousal, and the two can be easily confused for one another. *Is that a kettlebell in your pants or . . . wait . . . I don't think that's how that goes.* Even if you're already in a relationship, try working out together, as couples who do report higher levels of happiness.[15]

You'll occasionally be fired up to exercise, but that won't happen every day. Real commitment requires effort. Am I typically excited to get out of my warm bed at 6:00 a.m. to go for a run while it's cold and dark outside? Nope. But I know that I always regret it when I don't move during the day and that I feel great when I do. So I force myself to get up, put on clothes, and *go*. Getting out the door is always the hardest part, so I usually give myself a pep talk: "You just need to sweat. You don't have to work hard. You just need to move." Once I start, it's easy to keep it going, and I usually end up finding a rhythm and pushing myself after all.

Part of what separates those who get out the door or walk into the gym from those who don't is the *why*. Determine why working out is important to you, and then be prepared to remind yourself any time your built-in excuse generator starts producing content. And if all of your other *whys* fail, use whatever guilt you know you're going to feel as motivation. You don't have to do a ninety-minute routine of plyometrics complete with tire pulling, rope climbing, powerlifting, and knife throwing for it to count as exercise—all you have to do is break a sweat. Aim for twenty minutes. There will regularly be days when that's the absolute last thing you want to do, but it's essential to force yourself to cut the shit now and then. You might throw up the white flag occasionally (because sometimes the power of a warm bed is too strong), but chances are far greater that you'll win the long-term war with exercise if you know why you're fighting in the first place.

## When to Work Out

Working out will never just magically happen. It's a habit that takes time, which means you have to find a specific time for it.

*"I make exercise a part of my daily schedule. If I wake up in the morning thinking that I have to work out at some point during the day, I will plan my schedule around it. But if I only try to work out when I am not doing anything else, I rarely end up making it to the gym. For me, it has to be routine. It has to be as mandatory as anything else that I have to do during the day."*

—UNIVERSITY OF CALIFORNIA SANTA BARBARA, JUNIOR

One of the greatest double-edged swords in college is the schedule—or lack thereof. On the one hand, freedom is thrilling. I remember a semester where I only had one two-hour class on Tuesday. On the other hand, the vast amount of unscheduled time can result in zero daily structure. Some advice? Use this to your advantage and structure your day around exercise. You should have a lot of flexibility in regard to when you can work out because of the inconsistent schedule, which means you can play around with timing to find what works for you. Here are the two general time slots to consider:

*"The gym is a half mile away from my dorm, so I've started to schedule my workouts based on when I have class close to it. I'll wear workout clothes and then exercise once the class is over."*
—SARAH LAWRENCE COLLEGE, FRESHMAN

1. **In Between Classes.** If you have trouble motivating yourself to get to the gym in the morning or at night, consider working out before or after class. Your class commitments are usually two- to four-hour chunks spaced throughout the day, and exercise can be a great way to productively occupy those awkward periods of time that either fall in between classes, or between a class and your next meal at the dining hall.

   The time slot of your workout and its duration will likely change every day, depending on your class schedule, but mixing it up will prevent your routine from getting stale, and though you may have five different weekday schedules to keep in mind, your weekly one will probably remain the same for the semester (or quarter or trimester).

*"I work out whenever I have large gaps between classes. It helps to blow off some steam, and I always end up reenergized."*
—UNIVERSITY OF SOUTHERN CALIFORNIA, SOPHOMORE

When your class schedule does change, of course, you'll have to adjust when you exercise. Several students mentioned that they choose their classes strategically to create a block of time within each day for working out. Just a word of caution: when your schedule shifts, determine a new workout time ASAP. The longer you delay in adjusting your plan, the less likely you are to get back on track.

2.  **During the Daily Bookends.** If you're a creature of habit, you may opt to work out at the same time each day. There are two popular ways to do this: in the morning before class, and in the afternoon or evening after class. A perk of mornings, even though you may hate getting up, is that they are fairly predictable and usually free from last-minute social offers, unlike afternoons and evenings. Another perk is that the college gym is often *empty* in the morning, so if you're trying to avoid the meathead grunting Olympics, this is an excellent time to go. Pulling yourself out of bed can be hard, so mornings are easiest to stick to when you plan to meet a friend or attend a class, as both provide the accountability needed to whisper "not today motherfucker!" to the snooze button.

You might find, however, that you prefer to exercise in the afternoon or evening simply because it *feels* easier than moving in the a.m. There's some truth to this, as studies show that strength and flexibility are greatest in the afternoon due to heightened body temperature, and as a result, perceived exertion is low.[16] If you don't mind dealing with the crowds at the gym and don't find that your motivation dwindles throughout the day, this can be the perfect time to work out. Plus, moving will feel particularly great after a day spent sitting in class and doing homework.

> "I've started to exercise every other morning, and it has been the best decision I've ever made for my health. I lay out my clothes the night before. When I get up, I get dressed, put on my running shoes, and head straight to the gym. Even if it's just a twenty-minute run and some ab exercises, it's something, which makes me feel good."
> —GEORGETOWN UNIVERSITY, SOPHOMORE

Now, is there a really *best* time to work out? Yes. Whenever you'll do it! It certainly doesn't need to be at the same general time every day, and maybe a mix will suit you best. Exercise isn't mandatory, it doesn't have a due date, and you won't get in trouble if you skip it. Therefore, you need to set *yourself* up for success by tuning into your daily rhythms. Identify when you typically feel motivated and energized versus when you feel tired and groggy, and use that information in your planning. Only plan to exercise during windows where it feels doable, commit to showing up when the time comes, and then put in the effort to adjust when your schedule changes. Unless you're a college athlete, you won't have a coach who is going to get on your case for skipping practice. For exercise to happen, *you* need to make it feel important. Scheduling it into your day is the best way to do that.

> *"During my first semester, I ran regularly and was training to do a marathon. Unfortunately, toward the end of that semester, I got hit by the freshman plague. I was in bed for over a week. After that, my exercise schedule was never really a true schedule again. I got busy with classes shortly after that and never made time again. I still run every once in a while, but it is much more infrequent than I would like. I think that once you break a routine, it is super hard to get back into it."*
> —JOHNS HOPKINS UNIVERSITY, SOPHOMORE

The Normal Bar Survey, conducted in the mid-2000s, found that 30 percent of people cite lack of time as the reason they don't work out. Yet, 80 percent of those same respondents admitted to spending over an hour every day on the internet for fun.[17] The hard truth? You have thirty minutes you can devote to working out several times a week while still leaving time for everything else. If you're not willing to carve out that time, then it's not *time's* fault. You just don't want it badly enough. So go back to the last section and find a better *why*.

> *"There's only so much time in a day, and free time feels extremely minimal when factoring in class, homework, eating, and sleeping. In those free moments, I don't want to exercise. I'm tired, and I'm sick of doing things that I 'have' to do. I just want to relax and do nothing."*
> —UNIVERSITY OF SOUTHERN CALIFORNIA, SOPHOMORE

One of my favorite quotes for when I am feeling any self-pity about my lack of time for exercise is: "Someone busier than you is working out right now." I'm stupidly competitive, so when I think about all the people who are getting stronger while I'm making excuses, it serves as a wonderful kick in the ass. The bottom line is that taking care of yourself requires time, and exercise is a worthy investment of the minutes in your day.

## What to Do

The final piece of the exercise puzzle is figuring out *what* to do. Mapping out your workouts, just like you would your meals for the week, gives you purpose and direction when it's time to move. Pairing your *when* with a plan will increase the odds that you'll exercise.

I typically think out each week of workouts on Sunday, and this only takes a few minutes because most weeks look the same. There are certainly some weeks—hell, some months—where I don't actively plan at all and just wing it from day to day. But when I'm low on motivation or, conversely, hell-bent to reach a goal, I find that planning is critical. It's useful for three reasons. First, I start my week feeling empowered, as planning allows me to feel proud of my commitment to training. Second, I always have a workout "waiting" for me, so I don't need to spend time thinking about what to do when it's time to exercise. Third, the schedule holds me accountable. Without a plan, I'll skip workouts because I can just "do it tomorrow." I'm less likely to use that excuse if pushing things back one day throws off the entire schedule that I took time to make. Here are the five basic tenets of my workout plan, which are the same ideas I extend into the training plan I prepare for the athletes that I coach:

> *"You have time to hit the gym every day, it's just a matter of learning time management. It's crucial to learn how to schedule your day out."*
>
> —UNIVERSITY OF ROCHESTER, FRESHMAN

1. **Don't Go Too Big.** When I'm just getting back into training after taking a break, I have to remind myself to start slow. It's too easy to burn out quickly or get

injured when you don't correctly and gradually build up your fitness. If you're new to working out or haven't done it in a while, be patient. Treat it like climbing a ladder. You wouldn't try to jump from the bottom to the middle, because you're not a spider monkey and you'd probably smash your face on the rungs as you fell to your doom. You've got to start at the bottom and go one step at a time to safely get to the top. Progressing slowly can be frustrating when you're fired up to make changes, but take solace in the fact that your body will change simply by working out more than you used to. On the flip side, if you are overwhelmed day in and day out by the expectations that you are placing on yourself, you will quit. Both the frequency and duration of your workouts need to feel completely manageable, particularly in the beginning, so that you're always eager to answer the question "Where can I go from here?" rather than wondering, "When can I take a break?"

2.  **Incorporate a Mix of Easy and Hard.** Workouts should fall into one of two categories: easy or hard. An effective weekly plan should feature both kinds.

    Easy sessions should be low impact all around. They shouldn't stress your body or mind. Watch videos on your phone while pedaling on the stationary bike, go for an easy jog, or do abs with a friend. Easy workouts shouldn't be ones that you dread. They should feel like freebies, allowing you to cross exercise off your list for the day while challenging you very minimally. These days will enable you to recover physically and recharge mentally.

    Hard sessions should be the exact opposite. They're meant to be a little intimidating. They should provide a challenge and make you slightly nervous. Drag a friend along for these. They might scare you a little before you start—gearing up for hill repeats can make you feel like a small child surrounded by clowns in a horror circus—but they're the ones you'll be most proud of completing, and the only workouts you'll remember long after they're over. They're also the ones that will make you stronger, both physically and mentally. You only need to do one or two hard workouts each week to reap the benefits.

    Be thoughtful when deciding which days will be easy and hard. Consider your week. In the course of your Monday through Friday, you probably experience a mix of mellow and hectic schedules, and your workout plan should be based on that. Do you have a terrible Tuesday/Thursday class schedule? Then make those easy days or scheduled rest days. Just like the best time to work out is when you'll actually do it, the best workout plan is one you'll actually follow.

3. **Schedule Rest.** It's essential to give both your body and mind a complete break *at least* once a week. Use your scheduled workout time to sleep, do laundry, watch a movie, or cut those giant dirty hawk talons you call toenails. It doesn't matter what you do, as long as it feels restful and helps you recharge. Scheduled off days make it possible to maintain a regular exercise routine without experiencing burnout. Don't undervalue their importance, but also make sure that 99 percent of the time, your days off are planned and not impromptu. Looking forward to an upcoming day off will keep your workouts sharp and focused—giving in to excuses and allowing yourself to skip a workout at a moment's notice will not provide the same effect.

4. **Never Skip a Monday.** This is a simple exercise proverb that I try my best to honor. I've found that excusing myself from a Monday workout is like tripping at the starting line—I'm behind in my week before I even get going. I also find that when I skip a Monday, I end up eating like garbage during the day and not sleeping well, which sets a bad tone for the rest of the week. Avoid bailing on Monday by eating a good dinner, hydrating, and going to bed early on Sunday.

5. **Keep Things Interesting.** Not only is it boring to repeat the same workout every time you exercise, but it'll also prevent you from seeing gains. You wouldn't want to eat the same three meals every day because you'd get tired of the monotony and while also limiting yourself to a very specific set of nutrients, which could cause deficiencies in other areas. The same is true for working out. Incorporating variety is the easiest way to ensure that you don't tire of your exercise habit while also hitting an array of muscle groups and bodily systems. I alternate between two or three workout types—typically yoga, running, and strength training—to bring diversity into my weekly routine.

Once you've decided that you want to exercise in college, the world is your oyster. There are countless options to choose from, and most are paid for by your student fees, so they shouldn't cost you anything up front. However, the vastness can be overwhelming, particularly if you're just starting or getting back into exercise after a long break. To demystify your choices, let's walk through what you'll typically find on a college campus. As you're reading through these, keep a mental note of the ones that sound interesting so that you can work them into your plan.

## The Gym

Gyms can be scary. I had never been to a gym before college but got the impression after my first visit on campus that the cardio machines were to be used only by women in spandex, and the weight room was off-limits to anyone who wasn't sporting a bro tank and guzzling down liquid protein. On top of feeling self-conscious about not fitting in, I also had no idea what to do there.

> *"Gyms are intimidating. There are big muscular people there, and they're lifting hundreds of pounds at a time. It's not much of a confidence booster to go stand on a mat and lift your ten-pound weight while you've got grunting guys lifting weights twice your size."*
> —UNIVERSITY OF CALIFORNIA, LOS ANGELES, SOPHOMORE

If you're feeling that same way, you're not alone. According to one study, 65 percent of women and 35 percent of men have avoided the gym at some point due to fear.[18] Specifically, people are afraid of being judged by others for not being in shape or being inexperienced. I felt this way at the beginning, which is why I started going to the gym in my hometown before testing the waters at the one on campus. The environment there felt less threatening because most people were older than me and didn't seem remotely interested in what I was doing. Now, it's highly unlikely that the people in your college gym are looking at you and judging you, but if you feel nervous about that, getting some experience at a different location might help. If that's not an option because you're already in the middle of a semester, then ask a friend to go with you (there's power in numbers), go in the morning, and begin in the cardio room, as that's usually the least intimidating area of the gym. Once you've gained some confidence, spread your wings and check out the rest of the building. The college gym is loaded with options—give yourself a chance to explore them, if only for the sake of getting the most out of the two-thousand-dollar recreation fee you're paying with your tuition each year.

## The Cardio Room

The cardio room in any gym will be packed with machines for stationary movement—treadmills, ellipticals, rowers, stairs, and bikes. If you're brand new to these machines, the bike is an excellent place to start, then perhaps the elliptical or stairs. If you have experience running, check out the treadmill, and if you are willing to pay attention to the form suggestions on the side of the machine, try the rower. The great thing about using any of these machines is that you'll be in a temperature-controlled environment surrounded by cold water and TVs. You can go at whatever pace you desire and will be able to easily track your progress from week to week using the metrics displayed on the screen. Go with a friend, work out next to each other, and catch up while you break a sweat. Or go by yourself, pedal a bike, and a stream a show for thirty minutes so that you can cross exercise off your list.

*"You don't have to be a gym rat or start taking horse growth hormones, but try to get at least a half hour of cardio every day to keep yourself in check."*
—SANTA CLARA UNIVERSITY, RECENT GRAD

These machines are great for easy days, but also work well when you're ready for a good ass whooping. Interval training is my favorite thing to do on a stationary machine. Alternating between periods of work and rest is what defines an interval session. Essentially, you hammer hard for a manageable (and specified) chunk of time, recover, then hammer again.

The off periods provide a mental and physical break, and the on periods feel exciting, which makes interval training both engaging and effective. It's also much easier to monitor your form and work hard when you're only grinding for a few minutes at a time. Additionally, interval training is superefficient. A 2013 study found that twelve minutes of sprint-interval bike training done only three times per week produced the same benefits as forty to sixty minutes of moderate-intensity pedaling on the stationary bike five times per week.[19] You just earned back four hours! Interval training gives you much more bang for your buck than working at a steady pace. There's no better route for getting results in a short period of time.

---

### Sample 35-Minute Interval Workout

5-minute warm-up.

4 rounds of the following:

2 minutes at "moderate" intensity (challenging, but maintainable).

2 minutes at "hard" intensity (difficult to maintain, and hard to talk).

1 minute at "easy" intensity (relaxed, easy pace).

5 rounds of the following:

30 seconds at "hard" intensity.

30 seconds at "easy" intensity.

5-minute cooldown.

Total time: 35 minutes. To shift your intensity from easy to moderate to hard, increase your speed, the resistance/incline, or both.

---

## Fitness Classes

For some, attending a fitness class is less stressful than starting in the cardio room. You don't need to think in a class. You just have to show up and *do*. You'll have an instructor guiding you through the moves while demonstrating the proper technique. You'll also be surrounded by other people who're working hard, which ends up being a powerful motivator.

*"Our gym has ABT (abs, buns, and thighs), Zumba, spin, and yoga that all students can sign up for. When I am having difficulty getting motivated to work out, I force myself to do a class."*

—TULANE UNIVERSITY, JUNIOR

Plus, classes are typically an hour long, so if you have trouble forcing yourself to stay on an elliptical for that duration of time but are looking to add in longer workouts, this is an easy way to do that. I often use classes as my "hard" workouts because the nature of signing up keeps me from wimping out, and having other people there helps me push myself.

If you need another reason to check out classes, keep in mind that they won't be free after college. Once you're out, you should expect to pay between twenty and thirty bucks a pop. *Woof!* Capitalize on the access that you've got now and try different classes so you learn what you like. The standard offerings tend to be spinning, yoga, Pilates, TRX, HIIT (high-intensity interval training), barre, Zumba, and kickboxing, but for a complete list of the classes at your school, ask at the gym front desk or look on your college website.

*"I wish I had taken advantage of the FREE gym while I was in college. It was huge, clean, close, and had free classes. That's pretty much unheard of once you graduate."*
—UNIVERSITY OF VIRGINIA, RECENT GRAD

## Body-Weight Circuits

Typically, you're welcome to use the empty aerobics studios when classes aren't in session, and since these spaces often have mats, they're ideal spots for doing body-weight strength training circuits.

Strength training isn't solely for those who are trying to get ripped—it's great for everyone, particularly if you're trying to keep your weight in check. Here's why: your body is continually utilizing calories to power the basic functions that keep you alive—breathing, blood circulation, reparation and growth of cells, and regulation of hormones.[20] The number of calories used for those systems in a day, known as your resting metabolic rate, is related to your sex and age but can be altered based on your body composition. Muscle tissue requires more calories for upkeep than fat tissue, and strength training is an easy way to swap fat for muscle. So, in conclusion, pump a little iron, and you'll burn more calories every day just by being alive. Muscle tee and protein shake not required.

Effective muscle building doesn't have to utilize extra weight because, when moved properly, your own body can wipe you out in a hurry. Body-weight training should be the foundation of your strength routine, as it allows you to build endurance while also developing body awareness, improving coordination, and increasing joint mobility, all with a lower risk of injury than if you were tossing around dumbbells. You can add weighted exercises when ready. Still, body-weight moves should always be a mainstay in your exercise routine as both the variety and functionality will keep your training diverse and fitness well rounded. Training like this is also convenient as it can be done anywhere it's appropriate to sweat.

*"I hate going to the gym because it's always packed with people who take getting swole a lot more seriously than I do. Instead, I decided to take up running and started doing body-weight circuits in a nearby park."*
—UNIVERSITY OF SOUTHERN CALIFORNIA, SOPHOMORE

The best way to start is probably just to head to a floor mat at the end of an easy cardio session and try a few moves. Practice two or three different exercises at a time, shooting for anywhere between ten and thirty reps (or repetitions, which is one complete motion of an exercise) for moves that work your arms and legs. You can aim for a higher range of reps with core exercises, generally somewhere between twenty-five and one hundred, which should be equivalent to between thirty and sixty seconds. For cardio moves, the number of reps depends on the intensity of the exercise. For instance, you'll be able to crank out one hundred mountain climbers much more easily than one hundred burpees. Therefore, time is usually a better metric for those moves, so shoot for between thirty seconds and two minutes. Proper technique is far more important than hitting some arbitrary count, though, so as soon as fatigue begins preventing you from maintaining good posture, end your set. Then take as much rest as you need to feel ready to start again. Don't put pressure on yourself to hit particular times and counts as you're familiarizing yourself with these exercises, and have your phone with you so that you can google moves you're not entirely sure about.

Once you've explored the list of exercises, you may be interested in doing more structured (and challenging) strength workouts. One way to accomplish that is with a high-intensity interval training (HIIT) circuit. This is the secret sauce of those expensive quick-fix programs, but the magic formula is not complicated, and it doesn't need to cost you a dime. Here are the four basic rules of a HIIT circuit:

1. **Plan:** Pick two to three exercises for each muscle group.

2. **Work:** Do arm, leg, and core exercises for thirty to forty-five seconds each, and cardio exercises for sixty to ninety seconds, resting ten to fifteen seconds between exercises if needed. Quality is more important than quantity for every exercise, so move deliberately with excellent form and take mini rests between reps if needed to maintain that. Download a circuit or interval app to help you time each work/rest segment.

3. **Rest:** For one minute.

4. **Repeat:** Two more times.

---

### Sample HIIT Circuit

30 seconds of triceps dips.

30 seconds (per leg) of Bulgarian split squats.

30 seconds of windshield wipers.

30 seconds of plank.

30 seconds of squats, jumping every fifth.

30 seconds (per side) of crossover crunches.

60 seconds of side shuffle with touch.

60-second rest.

Repeat two more times.

Total time: 70 minutes, not including warm-up.

---

Another HIIT option is to do what's known as a Tabata workout, which is eight rounds of twenty seconds on, ten seconds off for a four-minute workout. Sounds easy, but I promise you'll be breathing hard and sweating in less time than it takes to watch a music video. Pick two or four exercises and cycle through them during the twenty second "on" portions. Rest for a full minute before beginning another Tabata circuit with the same or different exercises. One or two Tabata cycles is good enough for a beginner, whereas three or four will kick the ass of even the fittest gym rat.

# BODY-WEIGHT EXERCISES

| ARMS | CORE | LEGS | CARDIO |
|---|---|---|---|
| Tricep dips | Crunches | Walking lunges | Burpees (Half/Full) |
| Lateral shoulder flys | Crossover crunches | Side lunges | Mountain climbers |
| Push-ups | Ab bikes | Cross lunges | High knees |
| Diamond push-ups | Russian twists | Back squats | Plank jacks |
| Incline push-ups | Sit-ups | Sumo squats | Box jumps |
| **Spiderman push-ups** | **V-ups** | **Bulgarian split squats** | **Bench hops** |

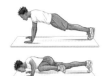 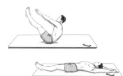    

| ARMS | CORE | LEGS | CARDIO |
|---|---|---|---|
| Inchworms | Leg raises | Chair step-ups | Squat jumps |
| Straight arm plank | Double leg circles | One-legged deadlifts | Frog jumps |
| Plank taps | Toe touches | Glute bridges | Lateral squat jumps |
| Plank walks | Dead bugs | Supermans | Lateral frog jumps |
| Side plank | Scissors | Side leg raises | Jump lunge |
| **Forearm plank** | **Windshield wipers** | **Donkey kicks** | **Knee jump tucks** |

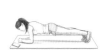 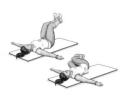 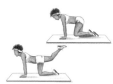 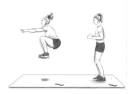

**Sample Tabata Circuit**

20 seconds of jump knee tucks.

10 seconds of rest.

20 seconds of spiderman push-ups.

10 seconds of rest.

20 seconds of squats.

10 seconds of rest.

20 seconds of bench hops.

10 seconds of rest.

Repeat.

Total time: 4 minutes; complete multiple cycles for a longer workout.

Body-weight strength circuits may start to get easier after you've been doing them for a few weeks. That means you're getting stronger! You'll need to increase the challenge to continue seeing gains, and you can do this by upping the time for each move, adding additional moves, decreasing your rest in between moves or sets, or tossing in some jump training. Typically, you'll need to make adjustments every four to six weeks. Cap any high-intensity workout at thirty minutes, not including the warm-up.

Don't forget to warm up before doing any of these strength training routines. Truthfully, I hate spending time on the warm-up, but it's stupid not to, as it puts you at a significant risk of pulling a muscle. Or worse. You might shit your pants! Well, that's probably only true if you drank too much the night before and haven't tested the movement waters yet. Regardless of the circumstances, always spend ten minutes jumping rope or running on a treadmill to work up a sweat *before* your workout to get your muscles warm.

## The Weight Room

When you're finally ready to face your fears of bro tanks, protein shakes, and power lifts, you'll be glad you did. Incorporating weights into parts of your strength routine is a surefire way to increase your muscle-building capacity and strengthen your tendons and ligaments. Not to mention that pushing and pulling some big, heavy plates can result in you feeling utterly badass. There are typically two areas in the weight room: one for machines and one for free weights.

## Weight Lifting Machines

My first foray into weighted strength training started with the machines, frankly, because it seemed like the safest place to begin. At my hometown gym, this is where the old people in Velcro shoes and old T-shirts hung out. Very unthreatening. It was perfect. Plus, there are directions on the side of every machine, and adjusting the weight load is as easy as moving a metal rod. Ideal!

Though a great place to start to get used to particular movements and build strength, there are also downsides to weight machines. Most gyms have just one or two of each, and they're often occupied when it's busy. *Bro, how are you still leg*

## WEIGHT LIFTING MACHINES WORTH A VISIT

| Lat pulldown | Seated leg curl | Seated chest press | Leg press |
|---|---|---|---|
| **SHOULDERS & BACK** | **HAMSTRINGS & CALVES** + GLUTES, QUADS | **CHEST** | **QUADS & HAMSTRINGS** + GLUTES |
| Keep back straight and core engaged | Keep back straight and core engaged | Plant feet on ground shoulder-width apart | Keep back straight and core engaged |
| Exhale while pulling bar down to top of chest | Position lower bar just below calves | Exhale and push out. Do not lock elbows | Exhale and push up. Do not lock knees |
| Pause, then slowly release while inhaling | Slowly curl while exhaling, hold, release and inhale | Pause at extension, and inhale while releasing | Pause at extension, and inhale while releasing |

*pressing?!* Additionally, these machines target a limited set of muscles and restrict your range of motion. Definitely start here and incorporate them into your workouts, but once you're ready, take the plunge and throw in some moves with free weights as well.

## Free Weights

When it finally became time for me to move on from the weightlifting machines, I gorilla-pounded my chest, roared like a warrior, stomped into the almighty freeweight room, and peed in the corner to mark my territory. *Step aside, Donnie! Those ten-pound dumbbells belong to me now.* There are three huge benefits to free weights. One, there are countless moves, so boredom is easy to avoid. Two, you can access a greater range of motion, allowing you to build strength that is both more diverse and functional. Three, since all that's required is weight, you don't have to be in a gym. You can get your own kettlebell or dumbbells and crank out sets when your roommates are gone, or when they're too preoccupied to notice that you're in the corner breathing heavily and sweating like a pig. *Don't mind me Barb, Tuesdays are for biceps.*

The one downside is that many moves are easy to do incorrectly, and you may need a spotter for some. To be absolutely certain that you're doing an exercise with proper form, it's best to ask a trainer at your gym. But since you probably won't do that, go watch a YouTube video or search for a detailed picture-driven tutorial online, then work out with a friend so that you can monitor each other.

Just as with body-weight circuits, you'll want to craft a plan before you start working out. For me, this part was particularly important in the beginning because it made the whole experience much less intimidating. Having a scripted workout removed the idle time I would have otherwise spent in between exercises aimlessly considering what to do next, and instead resulted in an efficiency that gave me confidence and made me feel like I belonged in the room. Here's a five-step how-to guide for creating your own workout:

1.  **Determine Routine Type:** If you plan to strength train once or twice a week, go for a full-body routine so that you hit all your muscle groups. More frequently

than that, and you'll want to consider doing what is called a split routine, where one day is arm day, the next is leg day, and then back again. When you lift heavy things, you cause little microscopic tears in your muscles. *Yikes.* That sounds gross, but the healing that follows is actually what makes you stronger. Healing, however, only happens with time. You're like Wolverine but with regular healing powers. So not actually like Wolverine at all. Taking a one- or two-day break from weights in between strength sessions is typically sufficient when you're doing a full-body routine, but if you want to strength train every day, then you'll need to alternate between muscle groups, hence the split routine suggestion. Allowing time for your muscles to heal will help you avoid overtraining and injury, both of which will ultimately cause you to lose strength.

2. **Select Exercises:** Six or eight exercises is typical for full-body routines, with an even split between arms and legs. Be careful not to get stuck doing the same six exercises every time you work out. Vary your moves so that you can build strength throughout your entire body. You can also include two or three additional abdominal exercises within your routine. Those would likely be done without weight, but if you're feeling crazy, use a medicine ball.

3. **Number of Reps:** The number of reps you'll do for each exercise depends largely on your intention. If you're looking to build overall strength, most resources recommend that you hit between eight and twelve reps per exercise. The heavier the weight, the fewer the reps, so those interested in powerlifting (i.e., getting bulked up) will likely only complete three to five reps of an exercise.

4. **Number of Sets:** Sets, alternatively known as rounds, refer to a group of consecutive reps. If you're performing eight or more reps, it's standard to do two or three sets. If you're a powerlifting beast, shoot for six sets instead.

5. **Amount of Weight:** When you first start training with weights, you'll need to do some data collection to figure out the proper load. For example, if you feel great using twenty pounds on the first of three sets of ten bicep curls, but can hardly make it through the sixth rep on the second set, back down your weight. A good rule of thumb is to start with what seems too easy

# EXERCISES WITH DUMBBELLS

| Upper Body | Lower Body |
|---|---|
| Wide grip bicep curls | Dumbbell swing throughs |
| Close grip bicep curls | Front squats |
| Bicep curls with overhead press | Split squats |
| **Front raises** | **Goblet squats** |

 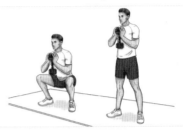

| Overhead presses | Front lunges |
|---|---|
| Bicep curls with overhead press | Back lunges |
| Bench press | Calf raises |
| **Skull crushers** | **Thrusters** |

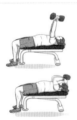 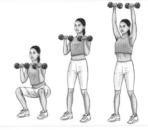

| Tricep extensions | Hamstring curls |
|---|---|
| Tricep kickbacks | Side squats |
| Hammer curls | Straight leg deadlifts |
| **Hammer curls with overhead press** | **Single leg deadlifts** |

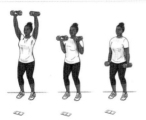 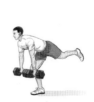 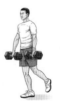

and build up. Get a small notebook or use the notes app on your phone to record how much weight you're lifting each time you work out (also document your reps and sets), and plan to increase the load as you get stronger. The goal with any strength exercise is to make it through each set without compromising form. It's okay for an exercise to become challenging during the last two or three reps of each set. You want those to be tough, as that's how you break down muscle to build strength. Just be mindful of your form; even one sloppy rep could result in injury. The mirrors in the gym are there so that you can monitor your form, not so you can check out your butt. *You know you've done it.*

---

### Sample Full-Body Weight Lifting Routine

Goblet squat x 10 (15 pounds).
Close grip bicep curls x 10 (15 pounds/arm).
Dumbbell thrusters x 12 (10 pounds/arm).
Hammer curls x 12 (10 pounds/arm).
Calf raises x 12 (15 pounds/arm).
Single arm dumbbell row x 10 (10 pounds/arm).
Repeat two more times.

---

Should you want some routine inspiration, there is no shortage of blogs, websites, and Instagram accounts that create and publish strength training workouts every day. Browse by googling or searching hashtags, find content that you like, and subscribe to their newsletter or feed. Even if you don't follow the workouts exactly, you'll see new moves that you might want to incorporate into your routine. Just be sure to trust your gut; if a move looks dangerous and dumb, chances are it is. You don't need to try everything you see.

There are also countless paid programs that will provide a thirty-, sixty-, or ninety-day training plan. If you prefer the ease of something premade and you have money to spend, these can be great tools. Plus, the training plans are yours forever once you pay, so you can repeat them as often as you like. I usually do one three-month strength training program each year, typically in the winter/spring when it's cold and I need motivation.

All right, enough talk of strength training! Let's leave the weight room, and head to . . .

## The Pool

Most schools have a legit lap pool, an amenity that becomes expensive and hard to find once you graduate. Swimming is the second most effective form of cardio after running, burning approximately three hundred calories per half hour. You can usually find your school's lap pool schedule online. Lousy swimmer? Same. I am no human fish, but I consider it a blessing because I can get completely wiped out in only thirty minutes of lap swimming. However, if you want to get better, some colleges offer swim lessons, PE classes in swim, or group water fitness classes. Interval workouts are great in the pool, but you can also go for a gentle swim on an easy day. Dominating in Marco Polo as a kid doesn't always translate to efficient swimming form, so ask someone who knows what they're doing for pointers if you need them. Having guidance to focus on will not only improve your swimming experience, but it'll also help pass the time while you're cranking out laps.

## The Track

If you want to do some running but find the treadmill as appealing as a hamster wheel, the track is a good alternative. Some schools have a small elevated track inside the gym. Bigger schools may have a field house with a larger indoor track, but if all else fails, your school will have an outdoor track somewhere on campus. Running can also be done around campus, or even out in your college town if that feels safe, but it's best to venture out once you've already built a baseline level of fitness and confidence.

**Basic Runner Safety.** If you're going to pound the roads or trails instead of the treadmill, observe these safety tips.

- **Run on the sidewalk.** If that's not an option, then run against traffic in the bike lane. The rules on trails are the same as if you were driving (in the US)—travel on the right and pass on the left.
- **Make eye contact** with drivers before crossing the street.
- **Don't wear headphones** during morning or evening runs, particularly if you're running in a secluded place. In fact, don't run in a secluded or dimly lit place. DANGER.
- **Run with someone** whenever possible, but if you have to go alone, text a roommate or friend and let them know where you're headed.
- **Bring your phone** so that you can access directions if you get lost or have the ability to call for help should you need it.
- **Trust your gut.** If a person or place seems creepy, don't be a dummy. Divert your course.
- **Check your weather app** before you go, and stick to the treadmill if it's hotter than 98.6 degrees outside with 70–80 percent humidity,[21] or conversely, snowy and icy on the roads. Extreme heat disrupts your body's ability to regulate temperature, and ice makes it difficult for drivers to stop and dangerous for you to run (google "girl falls running in snow video" for a good laugh and an understanding of why it's a bad idea).

I ran sprints in high school track. I didn't enjoy running and figured that was the most obvious way for it to be over quickly. I actually tried to do the shot put first—*zero running*—but my coach made me give it up after two weeks because I wasn't strong enough to pick up the ball convincingly, let alone throw it more than six feet, a distance that I think was a full ten feet short of what qualified as an attempt in New Hampshire high school track.

During my senior year of college, I was offered a job in California, teaching high school math and coaching cross-country. All I knew about cross-country was that it involved *a lot* of running—more than I'd ever done. My post–high school running experience consisted of two exceedingly pitiful 5Ks. In the first, I was beaten by an old man with a hunchback who was wheezing very audibly. In the second, I was beaten by *another* old man who was running with his dog. That dog stopped to take a dump in the middle of the race, he stopped to pick it up, and they both still beat me to the finish. My poor performances could have been due to lack of training or my assumption that prerace carbo-loading meant eating a deep-dish pizza cookie with three scoops of ice cream for dinner. Either way, the job was too good to pass up, and my role on the cross-country team seemed to be a part of the deal, so I made a decision: I was going to *learn* to run.

> "I used to hate exercise, but now it's a privilege I look forward too. I learned to run, and this past year, ran my first 5K. In the fall, I plan on running a 10K."
>
> —BROWN UNIVERSITY, SOPHOMORE

I was already in decent shape, so I took a big risk and signed up for a half marathon. I started by building a training plan, devouring as much information from books, magazines, and websites as I could. In the span of four months, I trained for and completed the race. I still got beat by tons of old men, but finished, and felt immense pride in that accomplishment. Though I was certainly no authority on running before I made it to California, I had a more definite sense of what it took to be a runner.

Discovering running changed my relationship with exercise. Once I got past the initial "I hate this because it's hard" phase, it became my favorite way to work out for several reasons. It doesn't take skill or experience to get started—just some interest, a desire to learn, and a touch of willpower. Here are five reasons running doesn't suck:

1. **Efficient.** Running burns four hundred calories per half hour on average, which is significantly more than any other form of cardio.
2. **Convenient.** Run alone or with a friend—anytime, anywhere, with almost no equipment. Running is an excellent form of social exercise because there's not much else to do but talk, which turns out to be a perfect way to make the time fly. You don't need fancy clothes, but you should run in good shoes. If you can

make a spiral with your shoe by holding the heel in one hand, the toe in the other, and twisting, it's time to upgrade. They'll typically cost you between $75 and $120, but they're worth the money, as good shoes prevent injuries.

3. **Goal-Oriented.** Races provide opportunities to set goals and measure progress. There are few other physical activities with such easy access to competition in adulthood. If you're cutthroat, you can start every race like I do—by covertly selecting an opponent after sizing up the other runners. *Great costume . . . now prepare to eat my dust.*

4. **Accessible.** You don't need any experience to become a runner. Nothing is stopping you from starting out with fifteen-minute miles that include regular walk breaks. Stick with it and continue to push yourself, and I assure you, you *will* improve. That alone makes running addicting—it's easy to track progress and see gains.

5. **Euphoric.** The runner's high is a real thing. It doesn't matter how fast you move, finding that magical mix of exhilaration and effortlessness after a prolonged period of running makes all of the pain worth it.

If you're starting at zero, do walk/run intervals a few times a week to get your body used to the impact. Once you feel comfortable, transition to continuous running at an easy pace for a short distance or duration. I still do runs like this once or twice a week for my easy days. If you'd like to continue getting faster and seeing gains, however, you'll need to work in some specific running workouts. Run training can be broken into three areas, which we'll call endurance, speed, and strength. These workouts can also be performed on a stationary bike, elliptical, or in a pool.

## Endurance

Being able to have a conversation while running is a good indicator that your effort level will be sustainable for a prolonged period of time. Medium and long runs at this pace will help you build up your endurance, which by definition is your ability to deal with "an unpleasant or difficult process or situation without giving way." You should be pretty tired and sweaty at the end of these runs, but not completely wiped out. Eventually, a distance that once felt hard will feel easy, which is proof that you can handle more, so gradually increase the challenge by adding mileage or increasing your time on the road to continue seeing improvements. Endurance runs are uncomplicated, which make them a great place to start with your training.

The mileage that constitutes an endurance run depends on where you're at. For those just starting, a range of two to four miles, alternating between running and walking, is probably ideal. If you are more experienced, your runs might be between five and seven miles for medium efforts, and between eight and twelve for longer ones. If you're moderately fit, shoot for four to eight miles when you go out. If you want to up the ante and keep things interesting on the shorter runs, finish with a fast last mile.

## Speed

Speed workouts are a superefficient way to improve your overall pace, torch calories, and reach the runner's high. That said, running fast might feel gross when you first try it. Nothing highlights sloppy mechanics like picking up your speed, and fatigue only makes it worse. However, your body will adapt with training, so be patient—you will eventually feel smooth and light on your feet.

A great way to start with speed is to try what is known as a "fartlek," which is a Swedish term that means "speed play." Take your medium run from before and toss in super-short bursts of speed throughout, with each burst being about twenty to sixty seconds. The "play" part is that the speed, duration, and frequency of the bursts are totally up to you. *Are we having fun yet!?* This is a perfect way to introduce fast running without any pressure.

When that feels manageable, consider trying a more structured speed workout. Hold a comfortably hard pace for a longer stretch, anywhere from two to ten minutes, then after each effort, recover with a few minutes of slow jogging. Repeat. These are known as tempo intervals, where "tempo" refers to the comfortably hard pace, and "intervals" explains the on/off nature of the workout. When you're ready for a more significant challenge, drop the rest and do a continuous tempo run instead.

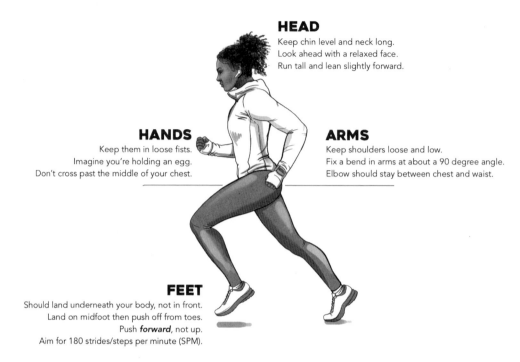

**HEAD**
Keep chin level and neck long.
Look ahead with a relaxed face.
Run tall and lean slightly forward.

**HANDS**
Keep them in loose fists.
Imagine you're holding an egg.
Don't cross past the middle of your chest.

**ARMS**
Keep shoulders loose and low.
Fix a bend in arms at about a 90 degree angle.
Elbow should stay between chest and waist.

**FEET**
Should land underneath your body, not in front.
Land on midfoot then push off from toes.
Push **forward**, not up.
Aim for 180 strides/steps per minute (SPM).

# RUNNING FORM

While there is no *wrong* way to run, the form that may feel most comfortable and natural for your body may not be the most efficient. Monitor your form by considering the four areas above. Even if they feel weird at first, all positive tweaks will eventually become second nature, help prevent injury, and make running easier on your body.

If you've never examined your running mechanics before, you should do that before you incorporate speed workouts. Running with bad form at any pace decreases your efficiency and ups your risk of injury, but it looks way worse when you're moving fast. So, have a friend who knows what they're doing watch you run and give you feedback. If that's not an option, have someone you trust not to make fun of you take a video while you run, then compare what you see to videos online. Of course, you're probably going to ignore all of this advice and skip the form analysis entirely, but it might be worth your time if you move like a wounded antelope.

## Strength

Fast running is more comfortable with strong legs, and there's nothing that will get your glutes, hamstrings, quads, and calves working quite like hill training. It's brutal but efficient. We live on a hill, so when I have limited time for a workout, I run up and down that thing as many times as I can in ten minutes. It's humbling how quickly it kicks my ass every time. Be sure to maintain good form—short quick steps with shoulders back and chest up—or your low back is going to hurt just as much as your legs when you're finished.

*"When I become overwhelmed, I make sure I give myself a break from my homework or the constant socialization by going on a run. I run off campus. I remove myself from the place of stress and get the reward of endorphins at the same time."*

—SCRIPPS UNIVERSITY, FRESHMAN

The process is easy: run up, recover down. You can sprint up short hills but will need to manage your pace more intentionally on long hills so your legs don't light on fire before reaching the top. If you can't find a hill, stairs work too. Use a back stairwell inside the gym, or head to the track and use the stadium risers if you have access.

You don't have to do a workout every time you run! Thirty minutes of gentle running is still an effective form of cardio, and once you get used to it, can be great exercise for "easy" days. For all of the workouts described in this section, it's important to understand when to call it a day. Once your form gets sloppy, or you're tapped for energy, you're no longer gaining fitness, you're just making it more difficult for your body to recover. Always stop when things become ugly.

If you find that you love running and want to try racing, there are tons of books and websites that offer specific training plans to prepare you for competition. You don't have to be fast to run in a race. In the past twelve years, I've run over eighty races and tried every distance from a 5K to a thirty-five-mile ultramarathon. I even did a half-Ironman once. Got destroyed. It doesn't matter how you perform, simply signing up will give you something to work toward for a chunk of time, as well as a way to measure your progress. Races provide a reason to stick to your training—a *why*. Racing can get expensive, but running is free and something that you won't have to stop when you go abroad, or worse, lose access to your campus gym forever. Speaking of which, let's talk about some other things that exist outside of the gym.

## Outside the Gym

Walking into the temple of fitness isn't the only way to get exercise on campus. I would suggest that you take full advantage of the options below simply because once you graduate, it'll be much harder to find organizations like these, particularly at low or zero cost.

### Clubs and Intramural Sports

Club sports are similar to high school sports, and often include tryouts, practice, and regular competition. By joining a team, you won't have to put much thought into what to do for exercise, and you'll have an instant group of friends. Most schools will have one or two club teams per sport.

*"I missed playing sports, so I joined the club volleyball team. It's been an easy way to stay in shape."*
—ST. MARY'S COLLEGE, SOPHOMORE

Intramural (IM) sports, on the other hand, require substantially less commitment. The chief obligation happens to be the best part of participating in sports: playing in games. IM sports leagues are typically tournament style: there will be a lot of teams who all play each other, and one will be crowned the champion at the end. *Fight to the death!* You can form your own team with a bunch of your friends or post yourself as a "free agent" and get picked up by a team.

*"To reduce stress, I used intramural sports as a way to give myself 'scheduled free time.' I forced all the people on my dorm floor to form soccer and basketball teams. It was hilarious. It was a disaster but in a good way. It was kind of like elementary school recess, except with more profanity. Twice a week for an hour, I could forget all of my classwork and assignments."*
—GEORGE WASHINGTON UNIVERSITY, FRESHMAN

There is typically a lot of overlap between what is offered at the club and intramural level. You'll see a mix of traditional sports (like what was offered in your high school) and less-traditional sports. Common offerings tend to be ski/snowboard, triathlon, running, lacrosse, rugby, badminton, racquetball, crew, Ultimate Frisbee, hockey, flag football, basketball, soccer, volleyball, water polo, tennis, swimming, fencing, cycling/mountain biking, taekwondo, dance, and golf. Don't be too shy to take advantage of the options. You may discover that you're surprisingly gifted with a sword—or you may just have fun trying new things with new people. For a complete list of what's offered at your campus, look on your school's website under the student life tab, or ask at the front desk of the gym.

## PE Classes

Most of the sports listed under club/IM are also offered as physical education classes, and there's no better way to make working out mandatory than to have it count for a credit or two. PE classes are a great way to learn the fundamentals of a sport, whether it's something you've played before or not. Introductory courses for sports don't exist in the real world if you're past the age of five,

> "Try something you've always thought was cool but were too afraid to start. I got involved in jiujitsu, one of my friends was on the rugby team, and another tried fencing."
> —JOHNS HOPKINS UNIVERSITY, RECENT GRAD

so this is another thing you shouldn't skip out on in college. Plus, with classes like self-defense, martial arts, backpacking, and survival skills, this could also be a great way to learn a sport or a skill that could up your uniqueness score and serve you well in the dating world, just like it did for me: "I got my degree in math. Oh, you hate math? Well, I also know jiujitsu and could kill you with a rear-naked choke. Do you still want my number?" Side note: I was never very good at dating.

## Walking to Class

If you're on a big campus, walking to class may fulfill some of your exercise quota each day. However, you may come to find that a leisurely stroll is not enough to keep you feeling fit.

If walking is all you have time for or all that you're physically ready to do, up the ante by walking at a brisk pace to get your heart working, and add some strength training to your day (even ten minutes of squats and push-ups in your dorm room is enough) so that your muscles get taxed. You can use a Fitbit, Apple Watch, or other step counter to keep track of how much you're walking. If you're using it as your sole form of exercise, shoot for fifteen to twenty thousand steps per day. If commuting to class doesn't help you reach your goal, go for a walk and call your parents or listen to a podcast to kill time.

*"For most of my first year, I defined exercise as my daily six- to eight-mile walk across and around campus. However, after noticing my body becoming squishy after just two quarters, I realized that I probably needed to actually work out."*

—UNIVERSITY OF CALIFORNIA, LOS ANGELES, FRESHMAN

## Crafting Your Own Workout Plan

Now that we've explored exercise options and the fundamentals of a good workout plan, it's time to make one for yourself! Below are several sample weeks to consider, designed based on specific goals. Each version features off days, easy days, workouts, strength training, and group classes or IM games. All of these plans *can* be completed in a gym setting, but certainly don't have to be. If you are comfortable running outside and doing body-weight strength sessions, you can take your workouts anywhere you want.

## Falling Off

I think it's fair to warn you that you will *not* always follow the plan you make, you will *not* always set aside the time, and you will *not* always listen to your *why*. Your intention to exercise will, without a shadow of a doubt, be called into question at some point. Things will continue to come up, or you'll find yourself repeatedly giving in to excuses. You'll get out of shape and be left with a choice: give up or get after it again?

## SAMPLE WEEKLY WORKOUT PLANS

| FOR WHEN: | MONDAY | TUESDAY | WEDNESDAY | THURSDAY | FRIDAY | SATURDAY | SUNDAY |
|---|---|---|---|---|---|---|---|
| *you're getting started* x 3/wk | **class or game\*** 45 minutes | Off | Off | **easy\*** 30 minutes | Off | **easy\*** 30 minutes **strength circuit** 20 minutes | Off |
| *you're busy* x 4/wk + 40 minute max | **workout\*** speed 20 minutes **strength circuit** 20 minutes | **easy\*** 15 minutes **workout\*** strength 20 minutes | Off | **easy\*** 20 minutes **strength circuit** 20 minutes | Off | **workout\*** endurance 40 minutes | Off |
| *it's almost spring break* x 5/wk | **class or game\*** 45 minutes | **workout\*** speed/strength 35 minutes **strength circuit** 20 minutes | Off | **workout\*** endurance 45 minutes | **easy\*** 30 minutes | **class or game\*** 60 minutes | Off |
| *you feel like a machine* x 6/wk | **workout\*** speed/strength 45 minutes | **easy\*** 30 minutes **strength circuit** 20 minutes | Off | **class or game\*** 45 minutes | **easy\*** 30 minutes | **workout\*** endurance 90 minutes | **stretch/ yoga** 60 minutes |

**easy\*** sessions should serve as active *recovery* and can be completed as a swim, run, bike, row, etc.
**workouts\*** are meant to be *challenging* sessions of swimming, running, cycling, rowing, etc. These be done as intervals/repeats or continuous efforts.
**class or game\*:** sign up for a fitness class or participate in a game for an intramural sport.

A lot of people give up. Remember, only 20 percent of American adults get enough exercise. Imagine how different that statistic would be if everyone who exercised clearly understood from the beginning that they were going to have to *restart* their routine eventually because that's just a part of the deal. It's the reality of health being fluid. The momentum you've built will, at some point, come to a halt for one reason or another. And that's okay. It's fine to take breaks. Just remember that you started to exercise because you decided it was important. And doable. And worth your time. You started because exercise plays a massive role in your health and happiness.

So when you take a break (or fall off the wagon entirely), and you want to get back, all you have to do it start again. Just start again. That's it. Knowing that you can *begin again* is what will separate you from everybody who throws in the towel for good. Starting over is a part of the process for people who prioritize their health, and giving up is the end of the story for those who aren't.

## How to Start Again

So once upon a time, you were in great shape, and now . . . not so much. Be easy on yourself and start light, almost like you're a beginner again. It might take a while to get your fitness back, though it's easier if you were in good condition before you took some time off. The important thing is to get started. You can't reach a goal if you don't begin moving toward it.

> *"I used to love working out, but things have gotten busy, and I've gotten lazy and have fallen off my routine. Now I dread working out because I am so out of shape."*
>
> —UNIVERSITY OF DALLAS, RECENT GRAD

The first day might feel great. You'll be fresh and fired up and almost surprised by how much fun you're having. Enjoy day one, because day two always sucks. *I'm too sore to even sit on the toilet.* The first week or two will be the worst, but know that it'll all feel better once the readjustment period is over. Your heart rate will no longer spike when you get started, and you'll get better at dissipating heat through sweat.[22] Stick with it for another two to four weeks, and you'll start to see changes in your body, which, if we're honest, is all most of us are waiting for. *Will all of this working out ever remove my newly acquired ice cream belly?* I get out of shape three or four times *each year* for one reason or another (vacation, lack of motivation, cold weather, Girl Scout Cookie season), and I promise: you will get your body back.

Any break less than a week long is negligible from a physiological standpoint, so don't stress when you miss just a few days. The key is to avoid breaks longer than two weeks. Regaining fitness requires more significant effort after this point, as you'll not only be retraining the muscles in your body but also the synapses in your brain. You'll essentially be starting from scratch, which is fine, just not ideal if you've been putting a lot of effort into establishing the habit.

## It's Worth It

I started working out as a sophomore in college, and it fundamentally changed me as a person over time. I found confidence in myself that I had never experienced as an athlete growing up. I believe this is because I was consciously deciding to spend time doing something hard because I knew it was good for me. That felt empowering, and still does—not everyone has the discipline to prioritize themselves in this way.

I didn't start working out to find that identity, however. My *why* was that I liked how exercise made me look and feel. Do I always look forward to working out? No. Do I follow my plan without fail? No. I'm not a fitness fanatic. I'm just a regular person who typically wants to eat chips, cuddle with my dog, and watch a movie instead. But I do my best to stick to the rules that I've laid out here, and as a result, have maintained an exercise habit for over a decade. Sticking to exercise isn't a complicated or magic formula. It doesn't require incredible willpower, great genes, or lots of time and money. All that's needed is a reason to begin, a sliver of time you can commit to, and a way of moving that you're excited about. Combine that with a willingness to start again when you need to that's free of self-pity and judgment, and you will be on your way to an exercise routine that will stay with you for the long haul.

## For When You Forget

Because friends, naps, homework, the weather, and "just not feeling it" can be powerful opponents in the fight for exercise. When you're ready to get moving again, start here:

- **Make Time for It.** Consider your weekly schedule and find a few windows that you can commit to. Avoid planning to work out at times where spontaneous snacks and appealing social offers could derail your plans, such as afternoons and evenings, especially on the weekend. Particularly when you're restarting, set your expectations for yourself at what feels more than doable. If you're someone who used to work out five or six days a week, then start back up again with four days and increase your commitment when you're ready.

- **Craft a Plan.** Exercising beyond high school sports means the responsibility of what to do falls on you. That ownership, however, doesn't have to be a burden. You have an insane number of options at your disposal in college and can incorporate as much variety and challenge into your weekly plan as you care to. Just consider your choices in tandem with your schedule at some point each week and map out how you're going to move. Establishing a daily plan will unquestionably strengthen your commitment to exercise. Do something fun and easy most of the time, but take on something hard once or twice each week. Above all, plan workouts that you're excited about, even if they scare you a little.

- **Generate Accountability.** Classes, clubs, teams, and friends make working out easier because they give you a reason to show up. Try to incorporate those things into your weekly plan as much as possible and use a watch that tracks your activity the rest of the time to hold yourself accountable.

Try to remember:

- **You'll Always Feel Good After You Exercise.** Especially when you don't want to. Exercise is one of the best tools we have for maintaining our health and happiness. It's simultaneously both protection and treatment. When stress is mounting, or you're feeling down, try taking a break to move. It doesn't have to be much, but breaking a sweat, pushing your muscles, and releasing some endorphins holds the power to change your mindset.

- **You're Going to "Fail."** Your commitment to exercise will most likely waver at multiple points each year, and that's entirely normal! Working out takes time and energy, and sometimes we can't or don't want to give up either of those things freely. Allow yourself the freedom to take breaks without judgment and get back to your routine when your resolve is renewed. It'll be easier to restart if your break was less than two weeks, but don't freak out if you're past that. Be realistic about your expectations in the beginning, prepare to suffer a little, and keep in mind that seeing progress and making gains can be an enjoyable part of restarting. Don't quit on yourself. You're going to crush it.

# CHAPTER 5
# STRESS

DAVE

**Growing up in a big city on the West Coast and choosing to attend a small college in the Midwest meant there were more than a few cultural discrepancies for me in my new surroundings.** The first person I talked to when I arrived on campus was my football coach, and the only thing I remember from our exchange was him making fun of my shoes. *You bring your skateboard, too?* Despite some very clear differences in clothing, musical taste, and hairstyles, my "fish out of water" experience was, frankly, pretty tame. I was a white male athlete with relatively good social skills at a school of primarily white kids. Playing a fall sport also made it easy to make fast friends and instantly feel like I was part of a community. Even with all of these chips on my side, I struggled mightily; making mistake after mistake, experiencing my first panic attack, and coming dangerously close to destroying my life. I had been flying high in high school and, basically, lit my wings on fire that first semester.

The campus security and local police kept a file of people to keep tabs on and annually updated the names every fall. I'd later learn that it took a whole two weeks for my name to make it to the top of the list. My first misdemeanor came when a cop walked into a bar, made eye contact with me as I was finishing a beer, and said, "You're Dave Henry, and you're not twenty-one. Come on, let's go." My roommate was my best friend from high school, and we'd both ventured to rural Iowa to play football and take over the school together. After partying every night for thirty con-secutive days, we got into a fight with each other outside of a bar and were tackled by two state troopers. He left the school shortly after that, and our relationship was forever changed.

I could never have predicted how traumatic my first year of college would be or the emotional toll it would take on my mental health. Depression and anxiety were foreign subjects, so I didn't really understand what I was feeling and didn't have the vocabulary to communicate it to someone else, let alone the courage. I found myself in a hopeless place where dealing with the world felt completely overwhelming.

Before we dive too deep into all the shitty choices I made and the bitter conse-quences they forced, I want to be clear about the intention for sharing my fuckups. I'm not suggesting you'll be a maniac like I was, and I doubt you'll endure the obstacles I unnecessarily placed in my path. It takes a rare breed of stupid to dig the holes that I dug, and I can own up to that wholeheartedly. What I can prom-ise you about *your* college experience is that you'll likely have to deal with more stress than you've ever encountered before, and the development of serious mental health issues is incredibly common. We all struggle with something. Whether it's the pressure of staying on top of your academics, getting into a nasty fight with your best friend, having a regrettable one-night stand, or trying to figure out how the hell you're going to pay for anything, the circumstances that can lead you to a dark place are numerous. The best defense you can have is knowing what to do when you get there.

*"There were definitely times when I curled up in a ball and refused to do anything but wallow in my own self-pity. It wasn't very helpful. One of the ways I managed stress on specific assignments was to stop doing work for thirty minutes and take a walk. Often I found a friend who was feeling stressed too, and we'd walk around for a little bit and either vent about what was stressing us out or talk about something completely unrelated. I realized that feeling overwhelmed and staying in my head wasn't productive."*

—GEORGE WASHINGTON UNIVERSITY, SENIOR

## Feeling Stuck

I love listening to music when I run. On top of tricking me into thinking I'm fast or turning the world into my own music video, it hides the less helpful thoughts that invade my brain. *I'm tired, I feel shitty. Why am I even doing this? Can I give up already?* You know, the usual. Even when I don't have music with me, I start songs in my head. Restart them when I lose my place. See how far I get with only memory to guide me. It's a fantastic distraction. *Hey look, just ran a mile.* When I get sick of the song, I change the station. Except when I can't. . . . *Damn you and your catchy hooks, Justin Bieber!* Stuck.

There will inevitably come a time when *you* get stuck in life, your feelings and emotions on repeat. With all of life's daily distractions, it'll be difficult sometimes to even recognize you're there. When you feel down, it can be completely consuming. Sadness and loneliness trapped under blankets of mounting pressure. The inner world caving in, the outer world turning a cold shoulder. *Sounds fun, right?* Frankly, that's been the scariest thing for me when I've been depressed: the idea that it will *always be like this.* Like I've entered a new "dark phase" of life that's relentless and unending, with seemingly no way out. Stuck.

Of course, all of this is happening between your ears. Recognizing *when* your mental health is taking a downward turn is the first step in figuring out *what* to do about it. This chapter is going to walk through how to recognize stress and deal with it when it hits. We're going to examine a few specific factors that have the potential to skyrocket your stress levels as a student and give you some pointers on how to get ahead of them. Stress-related conditions like anxiety and depression affect a huge segment of the college population, so we'll go over what the symptoms look and feel like when they arise, and most importantly, outline actions you can take to start feeling better. When you get stuck, this is how you can change the station.

## It Starts with Stress

Ever feel like the world turns you into a rage volcano? Where one bad thing leads to another, and before you know it, every stupid little comment you hear inflates your anger balloon until it pops and you explode hate bullets out of your eyes? Just me? Cool. While anger and aggression are not necessarily symptoms of stress, it's pretty common to find yourself in a situation where you think, *This shit . . . this shit right here . . . THIS is overwhelming.* You probably already have some understanding of *how* stress feels, and maybe you even can recognize *when* you're getting stressed, but you might not know from a hormonal level what's going on in your body. Goggles on, it's science time!

Stress is caused by a reaction to events that challenge the body or mind, called stressors. When you encounter a stressor, your body produces certain hormones to help you cope, which isn't necessarily a bad thing. If you stumbled across a bear in the woods, I'd hope your body would pump you full of *DANGER, WE COULD DIE* energy to help you deal with the situation. How else are you going to outrun your friends?!

Adrenaline is your "fight-or-flight" hormone. You'll feel it almost instantly when you're put in an exciting, threatening, dangerous, or stressful situation. Adrenaline readies you for battle—it speeds your heart rate, increases your blood pressure, brings tension to your body, and makes you hyperalert—all in a matter of seconds.[1] Basically, it's what superhero blood is comprised of.

The other stress hormone, cortisol, is a different beast. A much less sexy one. It's actually more like a vampire sloth that slowly sucks the life out of you. The release of cortisol is less evident because it's *slow.* It regulates your blood pressure, blood sugar, and fluid levels when you're stressed, which keeps your vital functions steadfastly operational, all of which sounds good. Unfortunately, it also suppresses your sex drive, digestive functions, need for sleep, and ability to fight off sickness.[2] Cortisol basically shuts down any system that isn't essential during battle. That's fine if you're trying to outrun a bear, but it's kind of annoying if you just have a paper due.

This entire grand hormonal design was created for dealing with short-term stress. However, one flaw in the system is that your body can *continuously* produce cortisol—even after a stressor is gone. If you're fixated on a problem—if you're stuck—you will steadily pump cortisol out, keeping many of your systems dulled down. That's when the effects of cortisol become problematic—an abundance of it in your system can be absolutely debilitating.

## Stress Management

When I'm overwhelmed by stress, the whole world has a darker tint. I can feel it everywhere, coursing through my blood. My chest gets tight, the muscles in my back tense up, my neck gets hot, and I clench my jaw. Negativity swirls through my mind, inevitably leaving me exhausted. It's pretty hard to do anything well under these conditions, which is precisely why it's so important to develop the skills to dig yourself out when you're in that space. Everyone needs these skills! Although stress sucks, it's an inevitable part of life, particularly for you as a college student.

According to the Spring 2019 National College Health Assessment, 98 percent of college students reported feeling stressed during the school year.[3] More shocking to me is that 2 percent reported not feeling *any* stress! How is that possible? Whether they're zenned-out teddy bears floating through life on velvet rainbows or secret serial killers that don't feel pain (or any other emotion), I'm jealous. At least, I think I am.

The more concerning statistics, however, are that 58 percent of students reported their stress to feel more serious than average, and 13 percent described it as "tremendous." Eighty-eight percent of students reported feeling "overwhelmed by all they had to do" at least once in the twelve months leading up to the survey, and 60 percent of those students had experienced that type of pressure within the last two weeks.[4] Stress in college is serious and, unfortunately, inevitable for most of us that have feelings.

*"Calling my mom, dad, or sister is always a good stress reliever, as is calling and catching up with one of my high school friends. For me, it helps to talk to people outside of the current world I am living in. It always feels like a breath of fresh air from whatever reality is stressing me out."*
—INDIANA UNIVERSITY, FRESHMAN

Since it's fair to assume that you're going to get punched in the gut by the swift fist of stress at some point, the best thing you can do is put a plan in place. Build your toolbox! A successful plan is twofold: it should include a handful of coping techniques for immediate use, as well as some stress-reducing habits that can be incorporated into your daily life. Having an action plan with your mental health is no different than planning your meals so that you eat well. Or deciding on a drink limit, so you don't vomit, shit your pants, and lose your shoes in the same night. Or mapping out your weekly exercise so that you actually move. It needs to be a part of your whole health puzzle. It deserves your attention. Don't overlook the importance of learning how to better cope with stress.

Everyone experiences stress differently, so you need to figure out what works for *you*. Start by paying attention when you're stressed. Work toward an understanding of what triggers you and what helps you deal. The suggestions we'll offer in this chapter are based on our experience, advice from our student survey, and the pros. Try some. Take note of which ones help, and start building your toolbox.

## Immediate Relief

When you realize that you're feeling overwhelmed, stop what you're doing. *Seriously, stop.* Press pause. Taking an uninterrupted moment to center yourself is often the last thing you want to do when you feel overwhelmed. *There's no time!* However, this reset is a critical first step in working through whatever is making you feel stuck and may actually reduce the total time you spend in that whirlwind of shitty emotions.

If you're standing up, go sit, and if you're in a place where you can lie down, then do that. Now, breathe. Really get into it. Make taking great breaths your job. Close your eyes, and take a long, slow, deep breath in. Hold for a moment. Then slowly release. Now do it again, but slower this time. Do it again. Try to relax your body. Are you doing it? When you're stressed, you'll have muscle groups working overtime everywhere. Could be your face, could be your shoulders, but you'll likely be holding on to something *somewhere* that you should let go. Breathing will bring release.

*"I manage stress by actively acknowledging when I need to take myself out of stressful situations. As someone with social anxiety, I've become far better at recognizing when I need to remove myself from an overly stimulating situation and be alone."*

—UNIVERSITY OF MICHIGAN, JUNIOR

Now it's time to drink some water. Every last organ in your body needs water to function. When you're stressed, your heart rate rises, and you breathe more heavily,

## BREATHING & RELAXATION TECHNIQUES FOR MANAGING STRESS

| | |
|---|---|
| **Basic Belly Breathing** | While lying down or sitting in a comfortable position, put one hand on your chest, and the other on your belly. Take a deep breath in through your nose, letting your belly rise but keeping your chest steady. Breathe out through pursed lips, using the hand on your belly to guide the air out. |
| **4-7-8 Breathing** | While in the basic belly breathing position, inhale through your nose for a count of four, hold for a count of seven, then slowly exhale for a count of eight. |
| **Progressive Muscle Relaxation** | While lying on a bed or floor, inhale for a count of four to ten while tensing one muscle group in your body (hands, quads, feet, shoulders, butt, forehead), then exhale for the same count while releasing tension. Lie still for a count of ten. Then repeat with the same muscle group or move to different one. |

and this can lead to dehydration. Dehydration is bad. When your water supply is low, your brain sends out an emergency "we're fucked!" call, which further increases cortisol production and adds to your stress![5] In short: stress brings on dehydration, and dehydration brings on *more* stress. It's a cruel joke.

Your thirst levels and pee color will help you decide if you're hydrated. Hint: having dry mouth and urine the color of caution tape *isn't* what you're shooting for. As a daily goal, you should aim to drink between half an ounce and an ounce of water for every pound you weigh. If you're 160 pounds, you'll want to shoot for between 80 and 160 ounces per day. You're not going to hit that goal by taking a slurp from the fountain every time you pass one or drinking an eight-ounce glass of water at meals. Go buy a bottle with a decent capacity, such as 30 ounces or greater, and carry that sucker with you everywhere. Fill it up when you enter the dining hall and again when you leave. Learn where else on campus you can refill. Water might not solve all your problems, but if you make hydrating a habit, it certainly won't be one of them.

While you are breathing and hydrating, you may realize that what you're stuck on isn't worth worrying about. There are countless small things that we *can* sweat, but don't *need* to. Do you remember everything that caused you to stress even two weeks ago? We tend to move past most of our stress without being fundamentally changed by whatever was causing it, so remind yourself that you hold the power to decide what's going to ruffle your feathers. If your stress really is justified, that's okay too. Relaxing your mind and body will eventually allow you to think more clearly and enable you to move toward a solution, which usually involves developing an action plan. Sometimes additional distance is required before you can make an action plan, so here are four resets to consider:

1. **Take a Walk.** Or go for a quick run, do push-ups, or scale a wall. Just move. From a chemical level, exercise is helpful because it triggers the production of endorphins, which immediately relieve pain and boost your mood. Studies have found that exercise not only reduces cortisol levels but also strengthens your resilience against future stressors.[6]

> *"I've found that rock climbing is a great way to de-stress during times of high workload. When I'm on the wall, all I'm thinking is,* Oh shit, I really, really don't want to fall. *All other problems seem irrelevant."*
>
> —SKIDMORE COLLEGE, SENIOR

From a practical level, permitting yourself some time to exercise gives you distance from the stressor, allowing you to clear your mind. Whenever I'm unsure of how to move forward with a problem, I go for a walk. I also mumble to myself about it, but that part's not necessary. I don't stop until I have a plan for my next few steps.

2. **Talk It Out.** When you first feel stress, whatever the trigger may be, you don't have to accept it at face value. It's so easy to twirl into a hate volcano when you feel like things are out of control. *I hate my professor! I hate this CLASS! I hate college. I HATE MYSELF!!!* Just because your *mind* tells you that everything is terrible doesn't mean you have to believe it. Pump the brakes long enough to have a conversation with yourself. Start to sort through what's overwhelming you until you can truly isolate the problem. You'll know when you've done that because pinpointing what's bothering you will bring the first wave of relief. Then consider possible solutions with a focus on your strengths. Be positive.

Forgive yourself. After you've done that, have conversations with other people who will remind you to do all those things again.

Rely on your support system when you're feeling overwhelmed. Call your parents, siblings, or a friend from high school. Vent to your roommate, a friend, your RA, or an adult on campus that you trust. Talk about what's dragging you down, or change the subject entirely. Shoot the shit, have a laugh—it doesn't matter. Socializing with others increases the "love hormone" oxytocin, which lowers cortisol.[7] This is why simply having a conversation, regardless of what it's about, can make you feel better. Pretty cool, right?

3. **Laugh.** Laughing isn't only way more fun than crying until you're dehydrated, screaming into a pillow, or staying eerily silent; studies have shown that it's a quick and effective way to reduce stress.[8] You physically *can't* feel anxious, angry, or sad while laughing because of the endorphins that are being released. I'm not talking about the nervous chuckle when the creepy kid compliments your yoga pants, I mean real guttural laughter, like when your best friend sneezes and accidentally farts in public. Listen to a comedy podcast, watch a funny video, hang out with friends who make you laugh, tickle your own feet with a giant feather—whatever works for you.

> *"Setting time aside specifically for goofing off is a part of how I manage stress."*
>
> —UNIVERSITY OF CHICAGO, RECENT GRAD

4. **Eat.** The first thing you'll want to eat when you're stressed will most likely *not* be a salad. Junk food of all kinds can absolutely seem like a solution to a wide variety of problems. The real kick in the dick is that food high in sodium and refined sugar (pretty much everything you'll be craving) actually increases cortisol production, which—get this—will only add to your stress! Boo! How messed up is that?

There are, however, certain foods (many of them are superfoods) that actually reduce the cortisol and adrenaline levels in your body. Dark chocolate is by far the most intriguing option, in my opinion, but the rest of the menu includes nuts, berries, oranges, oatmeal, spinach, salmon, and tea. My guess is that you're not going to whip up a salmon fillet in your dorm room, so maybe just keep some dark chocolate trail mix in a secret place. If you eat too much (of anything), it's still going to make you feel awful—but hey—at least you won't be stressed out about it.

## Long-Term Fixes

After some distance away from the stressor, it's time to start thinking about a solution if one is still needed. Some stressors go away on their own, but many others are simply problems that need to be worked out. In which case, it's finally time to make that plan. Don't skip this step. Avoidance is a commonly used coping technique among college students, as is shit-talking yourself, but neither one is ideal.[9] Avoidance merely slows you down, and beating yourself up will only make you feel worse.

*"This is going to sound corny as hell, but start by forgiving yourself for what you haven't done yet. Ninety percent of what kept me from doing what I needed to do was feeling angry at myself that I hadn't done it yet. It's okay, just start where you are and go from there. Also: there's an app called SelfControl that blocks internet access; it's a lifesaver. I felt like the biggest loser in the world, and also a millennial stereotype, while installing it, but I had to do what I had to do. Be honest with yourself about what you can't do or can't do well, and work around it. It's not the end of the world, it's just going to be hard. Set boundaries."*

**—NEW YORK UNIVERSITY, RECENT GRAD**

Your plan might involve making a to-do list, scheduling a meeting with a professor to get some help, apologizing to someone if you feel like you've messed up, getting more sleep, or simply just reevaluating your expectations. All that is required from you is an honest assessment of the situation and an ability to consider options. If you're struggling to think through those options on your own, enlist the help of a friend, sibling, parent, or therapist. The solution will always be different based on what's causing you stress, but the more frequently you view stress as a treatable problem that you have the power to solve, the better you'll get at knowing the right answer.

## Getting Ahead of Stress

A room filled with clutter will send Jill into a stress spiral. Actually, it's more like a tornado. She's not a fan of disorder and has a physical response to it. I definitely don't have this problem and could operate my whole existence in a mess without being bothered by it. But the tornado is strong, and I've learned it's best to be avoided. I'm a relatively clean person, but I'm not doing it for me. I do have my own triggers, though. When I deal with prolonged periods of physical discomfort, I have a tendency to turn into a poison-spewing hate dragon. I become irritable and overwhelmed by simple things. I've heard it's not a lot of fun to be around.

While the cause of stress will differ from person to person, the shitty feelings that accompany it are the same. Coping with regular stressors when they creep up is a skill that takes practice. The more you do it, the more natural it will become, and the negative impact that stress can have on your life will be minimized. However, research shows that embracing (rather than avoiding) the existence of stress, and then structuring your life so that you intentionally reduce stress whenever possible leads to . . . you guessed it: less stress.[10] Being proactive works. Here are three habits you can put in place at any time to reduce the amount of stress you expose yourself to in the first place.

1. **Do the Little Things.** The overarching themes of good health—namely, eat well, exercise, and get enough sleep—are important and can reduce stress, but establishing good patterns in all of these areas can feel ridiculously overwhelming when you already feel like garbage. So step away from the big picture and instead look for little tweaks you can make each day—either in those categories or other areas—to feel more in control of your well-being. Here are ten suggestions to get you started:

   - Make your bed.
   - Take a shower and brush your teeth.

*"I took a lot of time to be by myself in San Francisco exploring the city."*

—UNIVERSITY OF SAN FRANCISCO, RECENT GRAD

- Put on clean clothes for class.
- Eat a healthy breakfast.
- Plan your day.
- Take out the trash from your room.
- Drink a bottle of water.
- Put your phone on airplane mode.
- Make plans with someone.
- Go for a walk and listen to music.

Ultimately, it's about finding small, low-impact ways to take ownership over and improve the quality of your day. Do things that make you feel good. Things that you'll be proud of. The better you feel about how you're living right now, the more confident you'll be in your ability to make significant changes to your life if and when they're needed.

2. **Say No.** Your free time is a commodity that *you* ultimately control, so spend it in ways that serve you. That's not as selfish as it sounds. Okay, maybe it is, but who gives a shit? You have the right to be selfish when you're close to crossing your stress threshold. Put yourself first. Say no freely and confidently. Turn down commitments that will surely overextend you, don't occupy spaces that make you anxious, and stay away from people who piss you off. How you fill your days will impact your quality of life, so give yourself permission to be picky with your time.

*"You cannot do everything. I'm a very outgoing person, and I love being involved in activities at my school, but I overextend myself to the point of having panic attacks frequently. College is really fun, and there are so many opportunities to do things you love, but I think being able to say no to offers is a really important skill to have."*

—SARAH LAWRENCE COLLEGE, FRESHMAN

3. **Find Balance.** I know we've harped on this, but that's because it applies to every area of health. When you're in school, all play and no work will leave you without a job after graduation, but all work and no play may turn you into a sociopath. Neither outcome is awesome.

> *"My favorite stress reliever is clubbing because I've found that dancing with no inhibitions really just helps me relax."*
> —DURHAM UNIVERSITY, SENIOR

First, set aside time for work. *Really.* Treat homework and studying like a job, and find a multiple-hour block of time every weekday to take care of business. You'll always have work you can be doing, and by making a habit of reserving space for it in your day, you'll be in a better position to stay on top of it.

Additionally, set aside time every day for yourself. Do what *you* want to do, even if it's only for ten minutes. Free yourself from your phone so that you can enjoy life outside of the 6-x-3-inch rectangle for a second. Do something. Drink coffee, talk with friends, read a book, listen to music, or dance like an idiot. Honestly, do whatever it is that you like to do, just be sure that you give yourself permission to have some fun every single day.

> *"I mostly manage my stress by playing high-intensity video games that will demand my full attention. I know that this is probably looked down on by most professionals or whatever, but it works for me. It gives me a break from whatever is stressing me out and refuels me to get things done afterward."*
> —JOHNS HOPKINS UNIVERSITY, SOPHOMORE

## Communicate

Of all the things you can do to be proactive, learning how to talk about and process your feelings is the most important. This is one that will work for any type of stress because, remember, stress is caused by *your* response to a stressor. You are the first line of defense. This doesn't just refer to conversations with other people, in fact, a big part of this puzzle is learning how to talk to yourself.

*"Go easy on yourself. You're adjusting to a whole new environment—class-wise, people-wise, living on your own, making all your own choices, having to schedule your life, and to a certain degree, having to fend for yourself—it's one of the biggest changes you can make. So above all, you need to have your own back. If that means you need to have some cereal at the end of the day, take a nap, or skip going to the gym, then do it. Take an off day every once in a while. It's easy to get caught up in everyone else's way of doing things and to want to be like everyone else. But deep down, you are the only one who knows what you really want. You are the only one experiencing your life, so cut yourself a break if you need it."*

—UNIVERSITY OF SOUTHERN CALIFORNIA, SOPHOMORE

Be kind inside your head. Forgive yourself. You can't control how other people treat you, but you have complete autonomy over the way you treat yourself. That doesn't mean having constructive inner dialogue is easy. It takes practice to mediate yourself. To work on that, consider the following two options:

1.  **Journal.** Downloading your brain onto paper is an efficient way to start a conversation with yourself. There are no rules. You don't need full sentences or complete thoughts. Write about what's making you feel overwhelmed, angry, or sad, but also write about what's making you happy or grateful. You don't have to do this every single day, but getting your thoughts out of your head when you're overwhelmed allows you to sort through them, while also providing you with an opportunity to confront the most difficult ones head-on at your own speed. You don't need to use a traditional journal, either. You can write in your notes app, draft an email, or if you really want to share your feelings with the public, create a blog post. Don't like to write? Draw it out or make a video. Research suggests that the act of clearing your head, no matter the medium, is linked to a healthier mental state.[11,12]

**The Anatomy of a Gratitude Journal.** Research has found that unloading positive thoughts onto a page just three times each week is linked to an increase in happiness.[13] Essentially, focusing on the parts of your life that are awesome will make you feel less shitty. Most studies on gratitude journaling had participants cap their writing after fifteen minutes, but frankly, you don't even need to go that long. Keep a journal in your phone or a notebook, and make it a routine to write a few times a week after you get up, before you go to bed, or during any meals where you get the chance to eat by yourself. While there's no wrong way to do this type of writing, here are some ideas to get you started:

- **Consider a Range of Emotions.** Just because we're calling it a gratitude journal doesn't mean *that* particular emotion needs to be the singular one expressed on the page. Use these positive trigger words to get your brain firing: *Celebration. Fulfillment. Beauty. Appreciation. Kindness. Acknowledgment. Joy. Respect. Purpose. Laughter. Growth. Opportunity. Comfort. Inspiration. Freedom. Love. Wonder. Knowledge.*

  The main objective is to focus on the positive. If tallying up everything that's going well is proving difficult, flip your perspective and contemplate how your life would be different if you lacked certain blessings.

- **Praise Fellow Humans.** Instead of writing about *what* you are grateful for, write about *who* you are grateful for. Jot some lines down about the friend who sent you a funny GIF when you needed it most or the family member you recently had a great chat with. Research shows that when we witness or consider the kindness of others, we get a boost of happiness and feel inclined to be kind ourselves.[14]

- **But Don't Forget to Praise Yourself.** Using a gratitude journal to express pride in your own actions is an easy way to improve the relationship you have with yourself. If you took ownership of your day and kicked some serious ass as a result, it's okay to acknowledge how good that felt! Recognize your actions and affirm yourself! It will serve as a good reminder of what you're capable of and can help you shift the dialogue in your head from unsupportive to encouraging.[15]

- **Give Detail.** Giving yourself some time to sit with an idea allows for deeper reflection, so while it might be tempting to write, "I'm grateful for the weather today," take a moment to elaborate and explore the details. This doesn't have to result in significantly more writing, but considering specifics will extend the time spent in appreciation mode, which is the primary goal of this whole journaling exercise in the first place.

*"I started writing in a journal every night the summer before my freshman year. I've done it ever since. My rule was this: when I wrote, it wasn't necessary for me to write down every single thing that happened to me—or even to write about my day at all if I didn't feel like it. If all I felt like writing was the date and 'I'm tired,' that was enough. It's been really moving for me to be able to look back over my old journals—to remember fun and exciting things that happened, to see mention of the beginnings of things that would later become important, to be able to consider from some distance the way that I process the things that happen to me, and the patterns and paths that I follow as I grow."*

—YALE UNIVERSITY, RECENT GRAD

2. **Therapy.** One of the most efficient ways to improve how you process your thoughts, manage your stress, and care for any stress-related mental health issues is to talk to a therapist. Drop any stigma you feel, because there's nothing shameful about therapy. People go to personal trainers for guidance with exercise and dietitians for recommendations regarding food, right? Working with a therapist to learn about how you tick isn't all that different, and it's definitely a more interesting code to crack. Also, you don't need to go forever. A good therapist will help you set a clear goal that can take anywhere from several weeks to a year to meet, depending on which branch you end up exploring.

One type is cognitive behavioral therapy (CBT), an evidence-based practice that helps you examine the way you think, act, and feel. This is a great one to pursue if you need help controlling your inner dialogue and sorting through your feelings. Dialectical behavioral therapy (DBT) is a type of CBT that was developed to help people cope with extreme or unstable emotions and harmful behaviors (more on this later). There are many other types of therapy, but these are two of the most common.

A good therapist won't *just* listen to you talk, they'll work through your issues with you. They'll help you find solutions. They'll help you reframe. They'll teach you how to be kind to yourself. There is almost certainly a counseling center on your campus, and many schools offer free clinics. If you don't have access through your school, therapy is often covered through your health insurance. Even if you don't have health insurance, many therapists offer a sliding payment scale, so be sure to ask.

Be mindful that in the first few sessions, the counselor is just trying to get to know you, so don't give up on them too quickly. Many counselors who use CBT need to listen at first to understand how you frame your thoughts, and therefore, how your thoughts impact your actions. Be patient, as this can sometimes be a time-consuming process. That said, to make progress, you'll need to be with someone who makes you feel comfortable. It's worth taking the time to find that person, so know that you can switch therapists if the one you try first doesn't work for you.

*"If your school has mental health services, use them. If you're thinking, Oh, I'm just a little stressed and haven't been sleeping well, and I don't know what to do with my life and am scared all the time, but that's normal for a college student, so I don't need THERAPY, guess what? It is normal, and you do need therapy! You're setting a precedent for how your brain and heart are going to work as an adult human being—don't start off by white-knuckling yourself into a life you don't really want but don't feel like you have the tools to say no to."*

—NEW YORK UNIVERSITY, RECENT GRAD

## The Usual (Stress) Suspects

Preparing for the most common sources of stress—the shit that is inevitable—makes a lot of sense. Though everyone has a trigger list that is unique to them, college students tend to experience the most stress in four specific areas: academics, finances, intimate relationships, and sleep, according to the American College Health Assessment. We're going to walk through how you can be proactive to minimize stress in each of these areas, though we'll skip sleep for right now because we have an entire chapter on it coming up.

## School

Academics are the most significant stressor for college students, with 53 percent reporting that the pressure of schoolwork and maintaining a certain GPA has caused them trauma or has been very difficult to handle.[16] Overwhelming course loads, parental pressure, fear of failure, the looming job market, and the high demand of college assignments all contribute to that stress. Some legitimate ninja tricks can boost your productivity.

*"Having clear expectations of myself was important. I always wrote things down so that I could physically see what I had to do. It gave me better time management and kept my responsibilities from swirling around in ambiguity."*
—SEATTLE UNIVERSITY, RECENT GRAD

When you're having trouble dealing with the rigors of the college workload and all the other baggage that accompanies it, adopt the following three habits:

1. **Make a List.** Establishing a system for evaluating your workload is a critical first step in managing your academic stress. An easy way to accomplish this is to write down what you have to get done. This might be painful if the list is enormous, but downloading it from your brain gives you a chance to game plan. You can assign priority to the most pressing tasks and schedule blocks of time to take care of them.

**To-Do List Strategies.** To-do list creation and management is a skill of sorts. If you don't yet have a system that works for you, here is a process to try:

- **Weekly Overview:** Before the week starts, spend ten minutes wrapping your head around what's on the horizon. Record upcoming meetings, assignments (those that are due or require work), and personal tasks in the Notes app, a planner, or on a lined legal pad, organized by the appropriate header (appointments, school, and life). Not only will this give you an overview of the week ahead, it'll serve as a location to write down new tasks as they come up.
- **Daily Schedule:** Write out a plan for each day the night before or first thing in the morning. Start by blocking out time-specific commitments, like classes, work, and meals, and then fit flexible obligations, like homework sessions and exercise, in the gaps.
- **Task Sort:** Prioritize your daily schedule with items that are urgent (such as "due tomorrow") and important ("a third of your grade"). Tasks that are important, but not urgent, can be pushed. Further categorize tasks into small, medium, and large based on the brainpower and time required to complete each. The "1-3-5" rule suggests that a doable daily workload consists of one large, three medium, and five small tasks.

*"I'm a huge fan of to-do lists. My desk is full of Post-it notes, each for a different area of my life where I have to get things done. One of my greatest joys in life is taking a pen and crossing out one of my to-dos. I guess that's also a big part of how I manage stress. I don't procrastinate because it stresses me out more. When I get things done, the stress slowly fades bit by bit."*

—UNIVERSITY OF SOUTHERN CALIFORNIA, SOPHOMORE

2. **Capitalize on the Focus Windows.** Being strategic about *when* you sit down to do your work puts you in the company of some of the biggest ass-kickers in the

world. Biologically, people are wired to achieve peak alertness twice each day. The period of most intense focus comes in the morning, about two or three hours after rising, though we steadily become more alert from the very moment we wake up.[17] The other peak happens around dinnertime. Conversely, we struggle most with focus in the early afternoon hours, as concentration begins to wane after the morning peak, dropping to a low between 1:00 and 3:00 p.m. After that dip, it rises again in preparation for the evening peak, then decreases until it bottoms out in the final hours of the night, somewhere between 9:00 p.m. and midnight as we prepare to sleep. There's a hormonal justification for why you feel productive during some periods of the day and in a fog during others, as those windows are part of a predictable twenty-four-hour loop known as the circadian rhythm. The ability to capitalize on those focus windows can have exciting implications for your productivity. Mornings and early evenings should be reserved exclusively for challenging assignments, convoluted readings, and studying. In contrast, early afternoons and late nights should be used for work in less rigorous classes or simple tasks like returning emails and getting organized for the next day by making your to-do list.

Want to get even more strategic? Within every twenty-four-hour cycle, there are short, recurrent loops operating in the background that regulate energy output. These 90- to 120-minute cycles are broadly known as ultradian rhythms, though when it comes to human performance, many studies specifically call them basic rest-activity cycles (or BRACs). The two components are—wait for it—rest and activity. In general, the body and brain can only output energy (such as the energy needed to focus) for about 90 minutes before needing a roughly 20-minute break.[18] As we're nearing the end of a focus window, our brain sounds the "time's up!" alarm, which we consciously experience in the form of sudden urges, such as the desire to eat, drink, walk, nap, or check Instagram.[19] We fidget and get distracted for a reason—we're due for a physical, emotional, and mental renewal. While you may be inclined to ignore those impulses and push through the slump, don't. Extra energy is needed to pass the output limit, and it's supplied in the form of adrenaline and cortisol (remember those guys?!), meaning you're welcoming an imminent and unhelpful change in mood and increase in stress.[20] If you've been working for a while and then abruptly feel a shift in your ability to focus, take the hint! Set a timer for 20 minutes and leave your workstation. Go for a walk. Call your parents. Jump in the shower. Chat with a friend. Grab some food. Do a quick workout. Take a power nap. Once those 20 minutes are up, you'll be able to sit back down for another movie-length push with renewed resolve. And to achieve completely supercharged levels of focus during those 90- to 120-minute work bursts, you'll want to . . .

3. **Find the Flow.** Psychologist Mihaly Csikszentmihalyi is credited with discovering what is known as the flow state, which is "an optimal experience in which people are so involved in an activity that nothing else seems to matter."[21] The flow state makes time disappear, so it's basically a cheat code for humans to tap into other dimensional powers and kick unbelievable amounts of ass on tasks. This is where you can really become *super* you. If you've ever been so focused on something that you lost track of time and were genuinely surprised at how long you'd been doing it, you've probably entered a flow state.

How do you get there? First off, we're not fuckin' around. If you want the flow, you need to be serious! One requirement is that you have to have complete, unbroken focus to tap into the magical powers. So that means phone off or in airplane mode, email closed, bladder emptied, comfortable clothes on, and unhelpful browser windows shut down. If you need an extra line of defense against your impulse to break focus, download distraction blockers for your phone and computer. Establish a prework ritual. Get yourself set up with whatever drinks or snacks you need. Clean your workspace. Dab on an essential oil blend made to enhance concentration. Play some music through your earbuds—I personally dig instrumental movie soundtracks when I'm working. Do whatever is required to pump up your momentum and decrease the possibility of multitasking. The only thing you should be thinking about when it's time to work is the task you're about to dominate.

If you're someone who does better with small goals, you can break your 90- or 120-minute work session up into three or four 30-minute sessions, where you work for 25 minutes and break for 5—this is called the Pomodoro Technique. Set a watch or phone timer to keep yourself on schedule, and force

yourself to have laser focus during the work windows. Then you get to disconnect during your 5-minute break. Get a cup of coffee. Hit the restroom. Do
a breathing exercise. Stretch. Check your phone if you must, but stay away
from time sucks like email and social media. Once 5 minutes are up, set your
timer for another 25 minutes, and get back to work. Note distractions as they
come up, but do your best to push past them. It takes practice, but once you've
learned how to truly zero in, you should barely notice the time zipping by.
Eventually, you may be able to cut out the minibreaks altogether.

Another interesting flow requirement is that an assignment has to be
appropriately challenging. To reach peak engagement, you need to be working on something that is *just* a bit outside of your intellectual comfort zone,
while still having clear and reasonable expectations.[22] Before you sit down
to work, you should know exactly where you're going to start. Want to be
really on top of your shit? Read through assignments and brainstorm your
game plan the day or night before you plan to take care of business. If you're
not sure where to start and are freaked out because the assignment seems
too hard or you're confused about what's expected, take action immediately.
Email your professor for clarification, or get some insight from a classmate
or a TA. Figure out what is needed to fill in the gaps in your understanding
so that the challenge no longer exceeds your abilities, and most importantly,
*believe* that you will eventually be able to get it done. Avoiding a looming
task because it's difficult won't make it go away. So set yourself up for success
by staying organized, doing the hardest work during your peak concentration windows, and then putting your productivity on overdrive by entering
the flow state. There's no question that you will still encounter academic
stress, but it'll be much easier to manage if you learn how to engage with
your productivity superpowers.

## Money

It should come as no surprise that money is the number-two stressor for college students following academics, given that it's the number-one stressor for three-quarters
of the adult population in the US.[23] Chances are good that you've personally felt

the weight of financial pressures or seen them affect your parents. The price tag of college only exacerbates things.

College is insanely expensive. About 70 percent of students take out loans to cover the cost, with the average debt amounting to around $30,000 after graduation.[24] And while affording undergrad is an issue in and of itself, for the purposes of not getting sad and dark and talking about how crushing student loan debt can be, we're only going to talk about how to manage the financial side of day-to-day life on campus. Because on top of figuring out how to pay for tuition, food, and a place to live, you're going to need money for some things you need, such as books and transportation, and some things you want, like takeout and clothes.

Financial situations span quite a spectrum, and you will encounter people from all parts of it while you're in school. Some will have nothing, some will have everything, and some will fall in the middle. To keep yourself above water financially, it's important to set limits based on what you have, not what you're surrounded by. Take ownership of your finances. Granted, college plops you in a weird bubble of half freedom. You're living on your own, but probably not even close to being financially independent. You're becoming an adult, but can't work like one, and while you may not be burdened yet by the full expanse of "adult" expenses, you're still likely to spend some money every single day. To minimize stress and feel comfortable in your particular financial situation, you'll need to learn how to manage your money responsibly. Here are three strategies to get you started:

1.  **Earn It.** One surefire way to cut down on money stress is to make some of your own. According to the National Center for Education Statistics, more than 40 percent of full-time students work in some capacity during college, with the majority of that group putting in more than twenty hours per week.[25] On-campus jobs are perfect for meeting new people at your school, the commute couldn't be better, the shifts will accommodate your class schedule, the work is typically easy, and the weekly commitment is often low. For any on-campus job, you'll need to look at your school's website for postings, submit an application, and potentially interview. Expect to get paid around ten bucks per hour, and keep in mind that a typical semester is fifteen weeks, so if you're

working ten hours a week (which should feel manageable), you will rake in about $3,000 per academic year, before taxes.

If you have time for a slightly more substantial commitment, look off campus. While the pay is comparable to what you'd find on campus, the shifts are longer. Your school's website may have postings for off-campus positions, or you can look for jobs the old-fashioned way by putting feelers out to friends or strolling around town looking for "help wanted" signs. You'll have to interact with townies and leave your campus bubble, but honestly, that may be a welcome break, particularly as you near the end of your four years at school.

The most popular option, however, is working during the summer. Summer break is close to four months at most schools, so using that time to get a job and pad the old bank account can reduce or eliminate your need to work during the academic year. Even at ten bucks an hour, if you're able to get a full-time position working forty hours each week for the duration of the summer, you'd make over five grand before taxes. Look for work as a camp counselor, wedding caterer, babysitter, barista, ice cream scooper, house painter, landscaper, mover, paid intern . . . the list goes on. Plenty of businesses rely on college students for seasonal work. You've just got to find them. Plan to start your search between January and March for the best-paying jobs, and don't hesitate to look beyond your college town or where you grew up. Summer work can be a great way to explore the country (or world) and expand your network, which will become an invaluable asset for future jobs, particularly once you're out of school. If you're worried about where you're going to live, keep in mind that most camps and some internships provide housing, but even if that's not an option, subletting a room for a few months is usually an affordable alternative.

2. **Deal with It.** Some financial gurus say that you should pay off the interest on your student loan, begin a retirement account, or start accumulating a sizeable emergency fund while in college. Let's be real. You're not going to do that because you're not going to be making a lot of money. The financial goal you'll really want to focus on? Learning how to avoid overspending.

People have a tendency to tune out when they fear they've overspent because dealing with money isn't fun in the first place. Facing debt can be embarrassing and stressful. But money will only become *more* stressful if you close your eyes and hope that everything will be okay because you'll wake up one day and owe much more than you have. Which is a terrible feeling, by the way. It took me almost six years to pay off the personal debt I accumulated in college. I couldn't command much of a paycheck when I got out, and saving to pay off the debt was extremely challenging. On many occasions, my debit card was declined while buying groceries or gas. I'll never forget how that felt. While sometimes you might have to overextend in emergencies, creating a budget and tracking your expenses will help keep your finances in check.

You can create a super simple budget on a scrap of paper right now. The very first number to write down is the amount you can reliably expect to have access to each month. Whether this number comes from an allowance, a loan disbursement, or a paycheck, this *must* be your jumping-off point if the goal is to spend less than you make. Next, calculate the sum of your personal monthly bills, if you have any, and subtract that from your income. Then you should take out 10–15 percent of what remains because you *will* overspend at some point, and that little buffer will keep you from turning to your credit card. The rest is for you to spend, and you've got to make it last for the month. If it's easier for you to think short term, divide that total by 4.3 to get a weekly spending cap.

Setting the budget is the first step, but it doesn't do shit if you don't stick to it. If you'd like to allocate a certain amount for food or entertainment or clothing to hold yourself accountable, countless apps will help you to do that and then track your spending in each of those categories. Otherwise, you can just download a super simple expense tracker app to make sure you stay within your weekly limit, regardless of category. Budgeting and tracking don't have to be overwhelming or complicated, but it does need to happen. It's too easy to spend money when your debit and credit cards are hooked up to apps, websites, phones, and watches. Without a weekly or monthly limit in mind and a way to keep tabs on what you've shelled out, you put yourself in constant jeopardy of overspending. By regularly checking your bank and credit card accounts and monitoring your expenses, you'll not only increase your comfort and lower your stress when it comes to dealing with your finances,[26] but you'll also be able to halt any unintentional spending slides before they turn into full-on avalanches.

3.   **Manage Your Impulses.** *I really want this. In fact, I deserve this. I don't care what it costs, I'll put it on a credit card and figure out how to pay for it later.* Impulsive purchasing is easier than ever given the ease of paying with cards, and credit cards, in particular, make it possible to spend money on the things we want, even if we don't actually have the money to buy them. Over 30 percent of college students carry more than $1,000 in credit card debt.[27] Although some people use credit cards for emergency necessities, most debt is a result of impulse spending.

To minimize the frequency of your impulsive purchases, first, pull your card information off websites and apps. Make it a hassle to order takeout or buy clothes or other random shit through your phone. A slow payment process means you'll have to think as you're purchasing, thereby ensuring that your decision is not entirely impulsive. Second, have a sticky note near your desk, and when the urge to buy something hits, write it down. Once an item makes the list, wait at least three days before pulling the trigger. This will force you to think about how you're going to pay for it while also allowing you to assess how badly you want it. If you forget about it in three days, you can obviously wait to buy it or avoid spending that money altogether. The biggest burden of adulthood is having to deal with money. Learning how to budget and control your spending impulses *before* graduation will protect you from accumulating more substantial debt once the real force of adult bills start to hit.

## Sex and Relationships

Time for sex. Do I have your attention? Our intimate relationships can have a tremendous impact on our mental health, especially in college. How we interact with the people we let into our lives—the ones we get closest to—can be some of the most powerful influences on the way we feel. This isn't limited to just sexual relationships. A nasty fight with your best friend has the potential to wreck your week, or getting yelled at by your parents through the phone could send your head spinning. However, we tend to be even more affected by our romantic partners. Over a third of all college students have had a hard time handling an intimate relationship in the last year and have even described dealing with it as a traumatic experience.[28] *The good news?* There are some proactive steps you can take to help set your boundaries and expectations, both for other people *and* yourself. College is one big trial and error of setting your terms for interacting with other people. These are three basics to master:

1. **Communication.** One of the largest sources of stress in interpersonal relationships is not being on the same page with your partner. From establishing consent and methods of contraception to expressing your intentions and expectations, there's frankly a lot of stuff to talk about. As an adult, we respect your choices and only aim to help provide you with information to be safe and help you take care of yourself. We do believe you should save this type of connection for someone you care about, someone worthy, someone you'd be excited to have a conversation with the next day. Regardless of how you navigate your love life, if you decide that you are going get sexual with someone, it all begins with consent.

   While it may seem awkward, embarrassing, or even scary to say, establishing consent is arguably the most important conversation you can have with a sexual partner. It's an expression of trust and respect. *I trust that you will not make fun of me because I respect you too much to move forward without asking.* As we mentioned in the Booze chapter, consent is verbal confirmation exchanged between partners before any sexual contact takes place. "Do you want to have sex?" Yes/ No. It must be freely given, and all parties must feel it's okay to stop or say no at any given time. Just do it! Be scared and do it anyway, that's the definition of courage. By broaching something awkward and challenging together, you can actually become closer. And if the idea of talking about consent is stressing you out, it will pale in comparison to dealing with the consequences of *not* talking about consent. No one wants to wake up feeling like they were taken advantage of, or accused of sexual assault, or even worse. Avoid the pitfalls of ambiguity and clearly establish that you both are willing participants. If you can't have a conversation about consent, it's a good sign that maybe you shouldn't be getting intimate with that person, because there are other significant things you'll need to discuss, like STD testing and contraception.

By far the least sexy topic, sexually transmitted diseases (STDs) and sexually transmitted infections (STIs) are about as fun to think about as your parents having sex. Young adults (18–24) are more likely than any other demographic to participate in unprotected sex and have multiple sexual partners,[29] which, as you can imagine, puts them at the highest risk for contracting an STD. The most common STD or STI in the world is known as the human papillomavirus (HPV), which the Centers for Disease Control and Prevention estimates has infected seventy-nine million Americans and will be contracted by 80 percent of all sexually active people at some point in their lives.[30] There are over one hundred different strains of it. Though not all are high risk, some strains have cancer links and others cause genital warts. However, there is a vaccination for HPV that can be found at Planned Parenthood and other health clinics. Practicing safer sex with condoms is the widely recommended consensus by national health associations, as they can reduce the risk of contracting HPV and other STDs and STIs, including HIV, which still infects tens of thousands of people each year. Additionally, many schools offer free clinics where you can get tested and speak to a medical professional about all of this stuff. Is it fun to talk about these things? No! But it's an essential part of the package when it comes to your health. Having a conversation with your partner about getting tested for STDs and using contraception might seem like a chore at face value, but like establishing consent, it's an opportunity to communicate about something important and avoid even more stressful consequences of unprotected sex.

Discussing contraception is a responsibility that falls on the shoulders of both partners. If you are sexually active, talk to your doctor or other medical professionals about methods that will work for you. The most common method of contraception for women is still the pill, but there are alternatives, such as a birth control shot, birth control implantation, and IUDs. If you're not sure where to start or whom to talk to, your school's campus health services will be helpful in pointing you in the right direction.

Finally, what's your status? Are you exclusively dating? Is this a fling? While we're not suggesting there is a right or wrong answer to this question, it's no fun to be stuck in ambiguity. Get on the same page with your partner about both of your intentions to help clear up any confusion. Otherwise, it's impossible to set realistic expectations. It might be hard to start some of these conversations, but it's absolutely worth it. Be honest. Vulnerability is your superpower. If something is difficult to talk about, mention that it's difficult to talk about, but that you're going to try anyway. In my experience, people are inspired by expressing vulnerability and tend to meet your emotional level.

2. **Evaluating Your Relationship.** Our intimate relationships are powerful and can treat our feelings like an emotional punching bag at times. It's crucial to assess the impact a romantic relationship is having on your life. If it's a source of stress and anxiety, it might be best to move on. You're going to have your hands full balancing schoolwork, jobs, internships, your health, and your social life—make sure your partner proves to be worth the time and energy a relationship can consume. Here are some questions to ask yourself to understand the quality of your relationship better and whether or not it's having a positive effect on your life: *Do I feel respected and supported? Am I able to maintain relationships with other friends and family? Can we resolve conflict fairly? Am I able to express myself without fear of consequence? Do I feel like I have access to privacy? How does my partner make me feel about myself? Has my relationship affected my self-esteem?* If you think you are potentially in a toxic or abusive relationship, physically or emotionally, schedule an appointment at your student health center. Consulting some expert advice will give you the best guidance on how to proceed.

3. **Dealing with a Breakup.** Breakups are the fucking worst. All consuming and gut wrenching, they can feel like your entire world stops and all you can do is think about it over and over again. Dealing with it takes a healthy dose of processing, action, and, unfortunately, time. First and foremost, you need an outlet: someone you know and trust that you can talk to about your feelings. You've got a lot going on inside, and finding a healthy way to let it out will be to your benefit. Not only will talking it out provide a cathartic release, but it will also allow someone you know and trust to provide feedback. It's easier for people who are not swimming in the same swirling feelings to be objective about

the situation. A loss of a relationship is just that, a loss, and will most likely take some time to grieve the sudden change in your life. Just remember, you are also not alone in this grief, and it's arguably an essential part of the human experience. Everyone has heartbreak in their past, and in my experience, it's been a crucial part of learning and growing as a person. Try your best to learn from mistakes and refine your preferences as a result. Your list of "what I'm looking for in another person" can grow both from things you liked and didn't like about your last relationship. All the pain will pass with time. You got this!

The next step is to stay busy. Idle time can be your worst enemy when dealing with heartache. Rather than locking yourself in your room every night with your best friends Ben and Jerry, proactively make plans to do things that make you feel good. Because breakups tend to be a sudden change, this is a perfect opportunity to start some new healthy habits (we'll talk more about *how* in the Trial and Error chapter). Sign up for a club. Go see some live music. Start a new workout plan. Take a cooking class. Be active and do things that you enjoy doing. After all, you've just been given the gift of more time! Invest in yourself and pursue the interests that you find fascinating. Visit your student life center and see what your school has to offer. You're free! Go let some stress out, have some laughs, and discover that you're more resilient than you ever knew.

## Types of Stress

While we've been talking about coping with and planning for stress as a general thing, it's important to note that not all stress is created equal. There are two main types: acute and chronic. Being aware of which you're dealing with can give you a better understanding of the severity.

The less severe type is acute stress. Without a doubt, you've experienced this before—this is the stress you feel before a final exam or the night before a big paper is due, when you almost fall down a flight of stairs or nearly drop something fragile, or when you unexpectedly get spooked by a bug that's somewhere it's not supposed to be. *Spider!* It's easy to identify as it's usually related to an upcoming or recent event. In many instances, you may actually feel your body flood with hormones. The word *stress* typically has a negative connotation, but at certain times a little acute stress can actually be valuable. It gets you firing on all cylinders, which can help keep you safe in a shady situation or allow you to get shit done when you're feeling the pressure of a deadline.

Acute stress doesn't feel good in our bodies, but we're well equipped to handle it. It usually dissipates on its own with some distance from the stressor, either over time or by physically removing yourself from the source of your stress. Even if it lingers, it's manageable when dealt with promptly.

Too much acute stress, however, can be exhausting. Frequent or episodic acute stress is typically experienced by those who tend to have chaotic lives—often people who are overcommitted and disorganized.[31] The symptoms are mostly the same as regular acute stress, but the emotional toll it can take on the individual and those around them is more significant. Unfortunately, people who experience episodic acute stress often don't realize that there's anything wrong with how they're conducting their lives. They see their frenetic behavior as a part of their identity.

Dialectical behavioral therapy (DBT), which we mentioned earlier, was created precisely for dealing with these types of issues. When people suffer from episodic acute stress, they often need to put regular habits in place to prevent themselves from continuously engaging in stressful situations. Establishing those habits, however, can only happen when a person recognizes their stress level, typically with the assistance of a professional. If these symptoms seem familiar, please search for a DBT expert in your area and ask for a consultation.

Now for chronic stress. According to the American Psychological Association, chronic stress "is the stress of unrelenting demands and pressures for seemingly interminable periods of time." It's a kind of long-term stress caused by something which is a mainstay in your life—think a bad relationship, toxic living situation, or overwhelming academic responsibilities.

Chronic stress is problematic because your body doesn't get a chance to right itself if the stressor never dissipates. Your blood pressure and heart rate stay elevated. Your muscles remain tense. Your body has to work extra hard to continue functioning normally.[32] It sounds terrible because it is. Chronic stress can affect your personality, your health, your relationships—your entire life. Even worse, it's possible to live with and not recognize, as the stress can start to feel familiar.

If you believe that you are experiencing chronic stress, it's time to seek out help. Ignoring the problem will not make it go away. Conversely, things *will* get easier once you start working toward a solution. While that may require some significant changes to your life, you will be happier once the looming source of stress is removed. Look to your school's website for counseling information, or ask a friend or loved one to help you search for options. Chronic stress alone is challenging, but it can balloon into a more serious stress-related condition if left untreated.

## Stress-Related Conditions and Concerns

When stress goes unresolved and we carry it for prolonged periods of time, it can snowball into something more serious. Anxiety and depression are the two most common mental health obstacles that students encounter in college. Each year, about one in four students is treated by a professional for one of those two conditions, and 16 percent are treated for both.[33] Anxiety and depression are best addressed with the guidance of a mental health professional. Thankfully, acknowledging these and other mental health issues has become much less stigmatized in the last decade. The percentage of students turning to campus counseling centers for guidance has been rising steadily.

Between 2010 and 2015 alone, there was a 30 percent increase in the number of students seeking appointments with mental health counselors.[34] Many schools also offer stress assessment quizzes on their website, and several research universities are in the process of developing AI technology to identify and communicate with students who are at a high risk of stress and stress-related mental health issues. Schools are becoming increasingly aware that their students need support. Many campuses have free clinics that employ grad students. Your campus has resources, and you're paying to be there, so don't be afraid to use them. They're there for your benefit.

## Anxiety

Stress and anxiety are confusingly similar. In fact, feeling nervous or anxious is one of the symptoms of stress! There's quite an overlap in the physical symptoms, but unlike both chronic and acute stress—which are cued by a specific trigger or stressor—anxiety is stress that occurs without the presence of a stressor or continues long after the stressor has passed. Sixty-six percent of college students report feeling *overwhelming* anxiety at some point during the school year.[35] It's easy to find yourself nervously worrying over the multitude of uncertainties surrounding seemingly every decision. While occasional anxiety is no cause for concern, for some people, the crippling feeling becomes a routine part of every day and can get worse over time. When left untreated, this type of anxiety can affect every aspect of your life. If the symptoms become more substantial than the events that caused them, it's time to talk to a medical professional.

*"My mental health in college was the worst it has ever been. Despite taking very good care of myself physically—always exercising, eating healthy, and sleeping enough—my anxiety got much worse, and I experienced a few minor episodes of depression for the first time. I sought out counseling on campus, and it made a world of difference for me."*

—SANTA CLARA UNIVERSITY, SENIOR

## Depression

We all feel down from time to time. Sad, hopeless, irritable. When the feelings are unceasing nearly every day for at least two weeks straight, it can be a sign that you're depressed.[36]

If you find yourself here, you are not alone. Simply going to college is difficult to handle on some level for everyone, as evidenced by the fact that "changes in residence," "changing to a new school," and "taking on a loan" are three of the forty-three items (numbers thirty-two, thirty-three, and thirty-seven respectively) on the famous Holmes-Rahe Stress Inventory, a cataloging of life's most traumatic events that is meant to predict the likelihood of an upcoming dip in mental health. Living on campus can further fuel the sadness fire, as several lifestyle factors linked to depression, such as consumption of unhealthy foods, limited exercise, and insufficient sleep, are all commonplace.[37] Top that off with the fact that the average age for a first depressive episode is the late teens/early twenties.[38]

# STRESS & ANXIETY

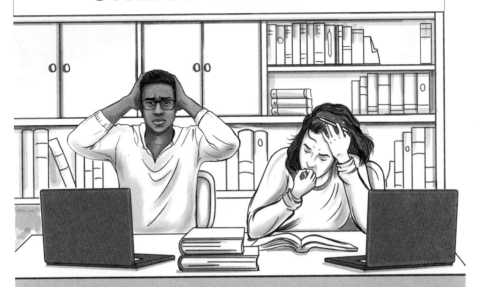

| ACUTE STRESS | CHRONIC STRESS | ANXIETY |
|---|---|---|
| Feeling angry, irritable, exhausted, or low on energy | Feeling isolated, detached, hopeless, or unhappy, feeling fragile, easily susceptible to crying | Panic, fear, or uneasiness, irritable, inability to stay calm, trouble sleeping, easily fatigued, muscle tension |
| Headaches or jaw aches due to increased tension in body | | |
| | Feeling like you have lost control of everything, difficulty sleeping, headaches and digestive problems | DURING A PANIC ATTACK: heart palpitations, sweating, trembling, trouble breathing (may feel like choking or being smothered), feelings of being out of control |
| Loss of appetite, rapid heart rate, shortness of breath, cold/sweaty palms | | |
| Exhibiting picking behavior | Thoughts of self-harm | |

symptom lists according to National Institute of Mental Health and American Psychological Association

This is not to scare you, but rather to explain that you're at an increased risk based on situational factors outside of your control. The good news is that depression is not a life sentence by any means—it's treatable! Keep an eye on your mental well-being, and if it feels like it's taking a turn toward something unfamiliar and unpleasant, don't blame yourself and certainly don't delay in getting some help. We tend to have an image of what depression looks like, but it takes many forms and affects people differently. There are, however, some common symptoms worth paying attention to listed on the next page.

If you find yourself nodding along to any of the items on either list, there is nothing to be ashamed of. You aren't the first to feel this way, and you certainly won't be the last. It just means it's probably time to consider talking to a therapist, counselor, or medical professional. On top of the instant relief you will get from communicating your feelings to another human being, they will also guide you through a slew of techniques designed to help you handle challenges on your own. They may even suggest that you take prescription medication, and if that's the route you end up going, there is no need to feel weird about it. If you had terrible eyesight, you wouldn't think twice about seeing a doctor for prescription glasses, right? A 2018 survey found that about 30 percent of students who suffer from anxiety, depression, or other mental health issues take medication, a number that has been steadily increasing over the past ten years.[39] While meds won't solve the underlying problems, they can be a wonderfully helpful part of a larger treatment plan. Bottom line? There are ways to feel better. There are trained people out there waiting to help you. It's literally their job to do that. Seeking out help isn't ever easy, but you will feel stronger and more in control simply by taking action.

All right, we're about to enter that last dark zone of the book. *You did it!* Even if you think this next section may not apply to you, please stick around for a touch longer. Spotting downward spirals is not only critically important for your own mental health but could also help you be there for others. You never know when you may find yourself in a position to make an enormous difference in someone else's life. Take a deep breath. Okay? Let's go.

# SIGNS OF DEPRESSION

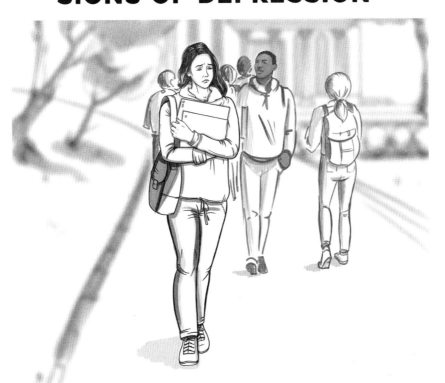

## MOOD & BEHAVIOR

feelings of worthlessness, emptiness, or guilt, loss of interest in activities, irritable, hopeless, persistently sad and/or anxious, difficulty concentrating, thoughts of death or suicide.

## BODY

decrease in energy, slow to move or talk, restless with difficulty sleeping (oversleeping or constant waking), change in appetite, muscle pain or headaches without clear explanation.

*symptom list according to National Institute of Mental Health*

## Suicide

> **Trigger Warning:** The next section discusses suicidal thoughts and tragedies that may cue intense emotional responses.

The morning after I got really drunk, free-climbed the facade of a large brick building, and threw blank CDs from a third-floor dorm room while chanting "THURSDAY!" over and over again, I found myself in quite a predicament. I forgot to mention that the CDs were flung via an open window of a third-floor dorm room that didn't belong to me. I also forgot to mention that later that night, the local police took me in for questioning and kept repeating the terms *breaking and entering, vandalism,* and *destruction of private property.* They told me I was going to jail for a long time. For hours, I vehemently denied it was me. When they finally let me leave, the sun was coming up. I walked home alone and stayed in bed all day, unable to sleep while awaiting two phone calls: one from the dean of students summoning me for expulsion, and one from the local police asking me to meet them outside. The phone never rang.

Sometime before dinner, I cracked. I could no longer handle my emotions, and I curled into a ball on the floor. I felt like my heart was going to explode. The pit of my stomach kept dropping into the falling feeling you experience on roller coasters. It took me another half an hour before I could pull myself together enough to call my parents. I told them I had just ruined my life and that I was probably going to jail for a while. I told them I was sorry and I told them I didn't know what to do.

It was the first time I'd ever thought about ending my life. *HOLY SHIT, I AM SO GRATEFUL I DIDN'T,* but let's get back to the *thoughts* part. Because I felt stuck in a bad place, it just seemed easier to disappear than continue the negative loop. I was overwhelmed with shame and regret. Only once I started to put my feelings into words and invited someone to listen was I able to let out what I had been bottling up.

Feeling the way I did is incredibly common—about one in seven college students has had suicidal thoughts.[40] I fell into that category, and I can't judge anyone's reason for why they felt the way that they did or continue to feel the way that they do. Suffering is suffering, regardless of circumstance—deep sadness does not discriminate and affects people in equally terrible ways.

It's incredibly rewarding to share your struggles. Aside from the almost-instant relief that can come from letting things out, it also allows you to get feedback. I can think of a few very powerful moments in my life where people important to me picked up the phone when I called. Sometimes they offered me advice. Sometimes they related to what I was going through. Sometimes they just listened. You are not alone in this world, and you don't need to feel ashamed if you've had dark thoughts as I have. Start building a list of people you can be completely honest with about your feelings. Include the counseling center at your school. Maybe you even include a church or chaplain's office. This does not have to be about making friends, it's about establishing a cathartic outlet for your emotions.

In a completely badass speech to Congress that saved funding for PBS in 1969, the great Fred Rogers said: "Anything that's human is mentionable, and anything that is mentionable can be more manageable. When we can talk about our feelings, they become less overwhelming, less upsetting, and less scary. The people we trust with that important talk can help us know that we are not alone."

We have to talk about these things. Not just on a personal level, but about how it is affecting our society as a whole. Behind car accidents, suicide is the second leading cause of death among college students.[41] More than a thousand college students take their own lives every year.[42] It would be reckless to claim a simple reason for *why* this tragedy is so common, but we can at least examine *what* you can do to increase your safety net. Under the Family Educational Rights and Privacy Act (FERPA), schools are not allowed to notify parents of serious academic issues. The idea is that college students should be treated as adults and given the autonomy to deal with their problems as they see fit. Universities can step in and reach out to parents only in a health or safety emergency, but in many cases, it can be too late.

In 2016, the *New York Times* ran a story about Graham Burton, who was a sophomore at Hamilton College when he took his life. His parents were completely blindsided by his death. While going through his personal items in his dorm, they were shocked to discover that members of the school faculty and administration were aware of Graham's mental health struggles and, in the case of some of his professors, had expressed their concerns to the dean of students. His parents couldn't understand why they hadn't been notified. The school, citing FERPA, offered that they were constrained from reaching out to protect Graham's privacy.[43]

*"It's very hard to spot depression. A close friend of mine was having a hard time at school and talking with professors in private, but never seemed sad. I should've listened better; we all should have. When we found out he wasn't studying abroad with us, and a teacher told us he was having a hard time, we didn't pay much mind to that because he was acting a little weird— not depressed, but just making uncomfortable jokes, distancing himself, and acting slightly out of character. Later he dropped out of school, then ultimately out of his third-story window in front of his father. Nineteen is far too young. If one of your friends seems off even in the slightest, sitting down with them in private and asking them if everything's all right, even if it doesn't seem like a big deal or that you're borderline pestering them, can save a life."*

—BOSTON UNIVERSITY, SENIOR

One thing you can do is sign a consent for your school to release records to your parents or emergency contacts. Now, this might not be a solution for everyone and should be avoided if it would cause more stress. You know your parents and have a better understanding of your relationship dynamics than anyone. As an adult, it's absolutely your decision to control your parents' access to your academic affairs. What you *should* consider is removing obstacles for others to help you. This may be as simple as passing your parents or loved ones' contact information on to a friend and asking them to reach out if they're ever worried about you. Surround yourself with positive people, and have a safety plan ready to put into place in difficult times.

I know all of this is heavy, but it's important. Hopefully, you'll never need to use any of this information, but if you do, it will always be here. Life is beautiful and challenging and absolutely worth sticking around for. Talk about your emotions, have a good cry when you need it, and make sure to be there for other people by asking questions and listening. Oh, and watch some puppy videos online. Especially the ones where there's a bunch of puppies running around and tripping over everything. Those are great.

> **Need Help?** If you or someone you know is considering suicide, the National Suicide Prevention Hotline is confidential and exists to provide support. Call 1-800-273-TALK for help or guidance. If you're worried that a friend may try to inflict self-harm, do not leave him or her alone. Call for backup, whether that's another friend or just someone else you trust to help. You shouldn't have to handle the situation on your own. Try to get your friend or loved one to seek immediate help from his or her doctor, campus security, the student health center, the nearest hospital emergency room, or call 911. Remove any access he or she may have to firearms or other potential tools for suicide, including medications. The important thing to remember is that contemplating suicide must always be taken seriously. You can't take the risk of assuming "they don't mean it, they're just venting, they're being dramatic." Let a qualified professional make that call.

## Don't Join the Contest

There's an unspoken contest that happens on college campuses all over the world. Anyone is welcome to join. The game is simple. The rules are clear. Overdo it. Take a full load of classes, pull regular all-nighters, max out your stress thermometer so that you can keep up with some set of expectations or demonstrate just how committed and serious you are about school. It's a contest with serious consequences. The worst part? No one wins. High levels of stress should be expected in college, given all of the changes you'll experience and the sheer amount of new responsibility you'll be handed. Don't get sucked into pushing yourself beyond reason. If you find yourself going down this road, all it takes to stop is your permission.

Mental health can be easy to ignore because it's not visible when we hop on the scale or look in the mirror. It's more like a storm cloud in the distance, waiting to sneak up on you with a torrential downpour. Don't let it. Don't allow dips in your

# WHEN YOU'RE FEELING OVERWHELMED...

- [ ] **Stop** what you're doing as soon as you start feeling extremely stressed or panicked.

- [ ] **Close your eyes** and take several slow **deep breaths** in and out through your mouth.

- [ ] **Repeat a mantra**, such as "I can do this," "this will pass," or "everything will be okay."

- [ ] Find an object to touch, smell, or taste - the **distraction** will help you shift gears.

- [ ] **Take a walk** and **listen to music** to clear your head and change your location.

- [ ] **Write** down what's overwhelming you or call a parent or friend and **talk** it out.

- [ ] If a solution to reducing your stress is clear, **make a plan and take action** when ready.

mental health to go undetected. Keep tabs on yourself and monitor your stress. Sometimes it'll resolve on its own, but other times you'll have to actually do something to deal with it. You might find yourself making jokes to take the edge off, but if you're really struggling, force yourself to have a serious conversation with someone. Tell your parents or a friend. Ask for help. There's nothing to be embarrassed about. There's nothing wrong with you. College *can* be really fucking hard, but it shouldn't feel unbearable. Being honest with yourself about the situation you're in and how you're coping is one of the best things you can do for your overall health and happiness. With an awareness of what feels manageable versus what feels like too much, I promise, you will be able to weather any storm that comes your way.

# For When You Forget

Because everyone gets swept up into life's wild stress tornado at some point. When you're ready to fight your way out, start here:

- **Be kind to yourself.** Feeling overwhelmed? Look to the basics. Go for a walk, take a shower, enjoy a delicious latte, eat a good meal, curl up for a nap, laugh, or have a lovely conversation with someone you like. Do the easy, small things that you know are good for your body and soul, as they will often end up calming your mind.
- **Communicate.** Stress can feel like one giant tangled knot in your stomach. The knot rarely comes undone on its own, so feeling better requires that you take the time to unwind it patiently. You might be able to work things out on your own by going through what's bothering you in your head or on paper. You might gain some clarity by talking to a parent or friend. Or you might need the guidance of someone with professional untangling training, like a therapist.
- **Be proactive.** School, money, and sex are three of the leading causes of stress among college students. Review the suggestions for kicking ass in those areas. Then pay attention to the other things that consistently stress you out and determine what you can do to avoid those triggers. Stress is all based on your reaction to stressors, so by getting ahead of what you know bothers you, you will reduce the frequency with which you feel stressed.

Try to remember:

- **Support your friends.** If you sense someone you know is acting off, ask them how they're doing and then listen. Help them sort through whatever puzzle they can't figure out, even if that only means suggesting that they seek out help. I promise you'll be glad you did. The interaction might not be incredibly profound, but it also *just* might.
- **Know the warning signs of serious stress-related conditions.** Checking yourself against the symptoms of chronic stress, anxiety disorder, and depression from time to time isn't a bad idea. Though many struggle with

these issues, it's believed that only 36 percent actually seek help,[44] likely because they're embarrassed to admit they need it or don't realize they have a problem. You should now understand that these problems are common, yet solvable, and there are people out there just waiting to help you out when you're ready. Trust your gut. You know yourself better than anyone else, so be your own best friend and advocate. You're worth it.

# CHAPTER 6
# SLEEP

---

### DAVE

**I've always struggled with sleep.** I have thousands of memories of lying in bed, tossing and turning, unable to shut off my brain or make my body comfortable. So naturally, my first night at college was an absolute nightmare. Mid-August in the midwest with no AC is one of the nine circles of hell. After sitting through hours of meetings and sweating through two separate football practices in sweltering humidity, when I finally hit the sack, I turned my pathetic excuse for a fan on high and placed it inches from my face. I continued to sweat as I lay awake for hours and pondered my life choices. I felt like my skin was crawling. Grabbing at my neck, I quickly flicked something into the middle of the room, jumped out of bed, and smashed it with my shoe. *That smell.* Only once my ears were away from the fan blades did I start to hear them. *All of them.*

No one knows exactly how the Asian lady beetle made its way to Iowa. It feeds on aphids and other insects on soybean farms in the summer, and come August, they make their way into unsuspecting homes. Sometimes by the hundreds. Covering entire sections of walls and emitting an offensive death odor when killed that I can only describe as a combination of melted plastic and old mustard. You know what gets me to this day? *Nobody told me about the fucking beetles!* I was around more than a hundred people on my first day of practice, and all of them forgot to mention that I might be visited by a biblical infestation of burnt-orange ladybug fucks. They bite too, or as an Iowa State professor so eloquently put it, "they will pinch your skin with their mouthparts." I killed at least fifty with a hammer before I realized I'd just fumigated my dorm room with toxic bug-guts. I didn't rest much during the late-summer beetle swarm, but my problems with sleep continued long after the cold weather pushed them south.

Sometimes I stayed up late because I was partying with friends. Other times because I was playing video games by myself. Mostly because I just didn't want to go to bed. I've always been a night owl, and more so than any other point in the day, that time felt like it belonged to me. Not having my parents around just made it easier to reinforce the habit. I remember many days feeling so tired I could fall asleep leaning up against a wall, and my 9:00 a.m. classes quickly turned into cruel chores. My sleep schedule was completely erratic, and I was tired all the time. It turns out, those are both symptoms of sleep deprivation.

> "Sleep, please. *I've only recently turned around my sleep schedule, but* wow. *It's amazing how much a couple more hours of sleep can make. Stress is inevitable, but finding a routine to minimize stress or manage it is absolutely necessary in college."*
> —SANTA CLARA UNIVERSITY, FRESHMAN

Scientists are still trying to figure out why, exactly, we need sleep. All organisms sleep, so they understand that it's essential and have studied the physical and mental repercussions that come from not getting enough of it.[1] Yet, there isn't consensus as to the precise purpose of sleep, a puzzle that is both frustrating and exciting to those in the field.

One thought is that the function of sleep is restorative. It allows our brain time to clean up the day's accumulation of a specific waste known as adenosine.[2] When we're awake, our cells are busy unpacking energy so it can be easily accessed by our body—adenosine is like the tossed-aside cardboard boxes the energy was packed in. It piles up throughout a day, and when enough of it attaches to the adenosine receptors in our brain, we get sleepy. That desire to sleep is a message to the body that it's time to tidy up and call it a day. It seems simple enough, but that's exactly the problem—scientists are confident that sleep serves multiple functions, and the sleepiness that adenosine brings about is just one piece of the puzzle. The one concept scientists are all certain about, however, is that insufficient sleep is a bad thing.

We're going to start this chapter by talking about why not sleeping enough, specifically as a college student, can be detrimental. Sleep is more complicated than "get eight hours." It involves considering your circadian rhythm, understanding the length of a typical sleep cycle, and creating the perfect hibernation zone in your dorm room.

## Downsides of Sleep Deprivation

Sleep is essential for our physical and mental well-being. It's also in short supply for college students across the country. Only 10 percent report getting enough shut-eye each night to feel rested in the morning,[3] which is a pretty significant dip from high school, where it's believed about 30 percent of students get adequate sleep.[4] Twenty percent report feeling sleepy or wiped out *six or seven* days of the week. It's nearly level with finances as the second-largest stressor for students behind academics, with almost 40 percent reporting that dealing with sleep has been difficult to handle or even traumatic.[5] Your body suffers on multiple fronts when you don't get enough sleep, especially in extreme circumstances. In 2014, a Chinese soccer fan died of sleep deprivation after attempting to stay up eleven nights in a row to watch the World Cup. *So crazy.* A lack of sleep will beat up your body, punch you in the brain, and make staying on top of your schoolwork nearly impossible. Sounds exciting, right? Let's dive in.

### Physical Repercussions

Feeling tired and sluggish when you're running low on sleep is typical, but there are a few other less obvious, yet more significant, physical repercussions that can come as a result of inadequate rest.

First, you'll be way more susceptible to sickness. While you're snoozing, your body produces little infection-fighting protein warriors known as cytokines.[6] You use an abundance of these guys when you've got an infection, inflammation, or even when you're battling stress. If you're not getting enough sleep, your cytokine

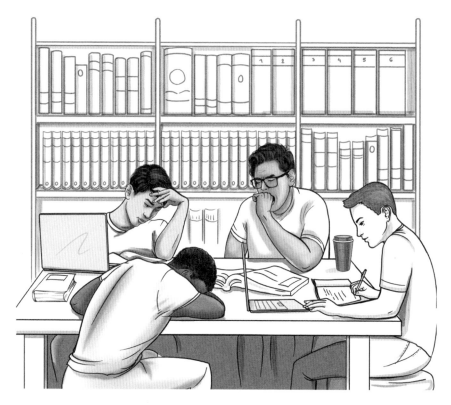

# THE FAMILIAR FACES
# OF SLEEP DEPRIVATION

production will be impaired, and thus, you'll be vulnerable to illness. You'll have a much better chance of escaping the powerful clutches of the annual college hell-plague with a shit ton of those bad boys on your side.

Second, you're at a higher risk of getting injured during exercise when you're sleep deprived. One study found that athletes regularly getting fewer than eight hours of sleep per night were 1.7 times more likely to get injured.[7] Even if you don't get hurt, you'll shortchange the benefits you receive from exercise, as your body repairs your muscles while you sleep. All those little microscopic tears that occur during training never get a chance to truly heal, meaning you'll miss out on attaining the Wolverine-like superstrength you should be gaining from your workouts.

Third, your weight can be impacted. Two specific hormones, leptin and ghrelin, get all out of whack when the body is running low on sleep. Leptin is in charge of communicating with your brain when you've had enough to eat, and ghrelin stimulates your appetite. When you're sleep deprived, shit hits the fan; leptin levels decrease, and ghrelin levels increase. In other words, your appetite will be raging because of the increased ghrelin, and your mind will be screaming, "*FOOD! MORE FOOD!*"—even when you're not hungry—because there's not enough leptin to shut you down.[8] If you're trying really hard to be mindful about your nutrition, but seem to keep losing control, inadequate sleep may be part of the problem.

However, all those physical drawbacks pale in comparison to the next one. It turns out sleep deprivation is *crazy* bad for your brain. Ready to have your mind melted? A sleep-deprivation study conducted on mice, published in the *Journal of Neuroscience* in May 2017, had a conclusion that made for a pretty insane headline: your brain eats itself when you're sleep deprived.[9] *Uhhhh . . . come again?* As stated earlier, the brain does a lot of housekeeping while we're sleeping. Which is a good thing . . . until we're really sleep deprived. Researchers were shocked to observe that the brains of those sleep-deprived mice went on a cleaning tear when they finally had a chance, clearing out the bad stuff, but also destroying some of the perfectly healthy, fully functioning parts! This would be like cleaning your dorm room and throwing your laptop and phone out with the trash because you were in a frenzy. *Don't need 'em!* Further studies are needed to assess the impact on the human brain. Still, this finding suggests that sleep deprivation can cause irreversible damage and increase the risk of Alzheimer's and other types of dementia.[10] So that's pretty terrifying.

## Mental Repercussions

In addition to physically feeling like a trash fire, not enough sleep can put you in a sour mood. When your sleep deficit reaches the level of chronic deprivation—insufficient sleep over an extended period of time (often cited to be about two weeks)—you will be *the worst* version of yourself: a big muddied mix of angry, sad, stressed, and overwhelmed. Sleep should be one of the first elements of your health that you consider if you're in a crap mood regularly and can't figure out why.

Sleep and mental health have a complicated relationship. On the one hand, people who suffer from stress and stress-related mental health issues often have more trouble sleeping than those who don't. Chronic sleep problems affect between 50 to 80 percent of patients seeking treatment for mental health issues, compared to 10–18 percent of all others.[11] The 2013 Stress in America study conducted by the American Psychological Association found that 49 percent of adults and 43 percent of teens report that stress causes them to lie awake at night. When short on sleep, 45 percent of those with high-stress levels (eight, nine, or ten out of ten) report feeling more stressed.[12]

*"Everyone talks about the 'Freshman 15,' so that was my biggest health concern going into school. My weight fluctuated in both directions during college, and the only time it reached an unhealthy point was in the underweight direction, not overweight. I was so anxious and stressed that I didn't eat or sleep for two weeks. I wish I was joking. When at its worst, I literally did not sleep for two weeks because I'd wake up with panic attacks anytime I closed my eyes."*

—UNIVERSITY OF ARIZONA, RECENT GRAD

While some doctors view sleep issues as a *symptom* of many mental health conditions, new research suggests that lack of sleep may actually "raise the risk for, and even directly contribute to, the development of some psychiatric disorders."[13] Regardless of which causes the other, a relationship clearly exists. Prioritizing sleep may protect your mental health.

## Academic Repercussions

Twenty-four percent of college students believe that their academic performance has been negatively impacted by inadequate sleep.[14] When you're tired, certain parts of your brain basically throw in the towel—specifically, your memory, cognition, and concentration. That's why a paper you write at 3:00 a.m. might read the next day like incoherent garbage. Impaired memory makes it difficult to file away new ideas and retain old ones. Focusing on a lecture is much more challenging when your concentration is jeopardized, and that's assuming you even make it to class. It's much easier to sleep right through your alarm when you're sleep deprived. Also, forget about tackling any assignment that requires critical thinking or logical reasoning while you're tired, as your problem-solving abilities will be on par with a sloth. Regardless of your major, whether you're reading a ton in a humanities discipline or doing hours of calculations that require precision in a math or science, you're pretty much guaranteed to do subpar work.

All of this can hurt your grades. One study from 2001 found a significant difference between the average GPAs of those who got more than nine hours of sleep (3.24), and those who got fewer than six hours (2.74).[15] Even those who slept between seven and eight hours had a higher GPA of 3.01. These significant discrepancies could get in the way of opportunities, like nabbing valuable internships or gaining admission to special programs. By not getting enough sleep, you are effectively undercutting your potential.

*"I'm proud of my ability to sleep enough. I've found that staying up late does not lead me to put forth better work. My productivity declines as it gets later into the night."*
—HAMILTON COLLEGE, JUNIOR

So, to recap. Without adequate sleep, you will be sick, weak, grumpy, and hungry (but not really . . . you'll just think you are), and your brain will be too busy eating itself to focus on your assignments. If any of those repercussions sound more like symptoms to you, that could mean you're already chronically sleep deprived. Not to worry! Sleep deprivation can be fixed, as well as avoided. Let's first discuss what "enough" sleep looks like and how you can go about getting it.

## Cycles, Rhythms, and Schedules

Understanding what happens when your head hits the pillow can be a difference-maker in your attempt to troubleshoot or avoid sleep issues altogether, so here we go. Sleep occurs in cycles that are between 90 and 120 minutes long, which play on repeat while you're snoozing. Once one cycle ends, you may or may not wake up briefly before immediately starting another. If that all sounds familiar, it's because sleep cycles are ultradian rhythms, just like the basic rest-activity cycles that we talked about in the last chapter. Activity in this context is the body undergoing repairs. Each sleep cycle has four distinct phases. The first three of those are different levels of non-REM or NREM sleep, and the last phase is the one you're probably most familiar with, which is REM (rapid eye movement) sleep.

The very first part of a sleep cycle, known as NREM Stage 1, is where you drift off. This period between wake and rest is fragile because it's easy to be woken up during this time. You'll be particularly sensitive to noise and light, but if you can

# A (SAMPLE) NIGHT OF SLEEP

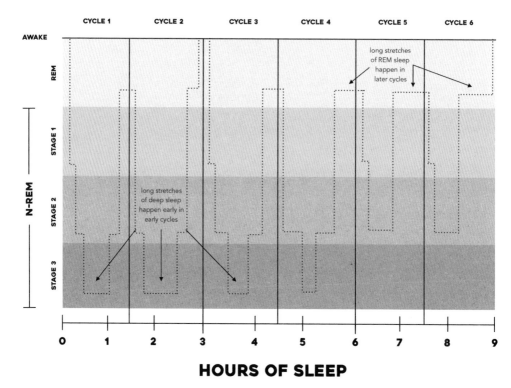

get yourself into a comfortable position and remove distractions, you'll typically transition to the next phase within five to ten minutes.

NREM Stage 2 is about twenty minutes long. This is where your body prepares for the deep reparative sleep that is coming by slowing your heart rate, relaxing your muscles, and decreasing your body temperature. It's still light sleep, so your roommate laughing at cat videos could wake you up and send you back to the beginning. However, you'll actually feel rested and refreshed if you wake up between NREM Stage 2 and NREM Stage 3. According to a NASA study from 1995, twenty-six minutes is the ideal length for a power nap because it keeps you in that sweet spot. These naps created super astronauts, boosting performance by 34 percent and alertness by 54 percent.[16]

Next up is deep sleep, or NREM Stage 3—the most critical part of the whole cycle. It's the mother of all recovery. You basically go into hibernation. *Do not disturb the sleeping bear!* If you've ever woken up from a nap super cranky and somehow more tired, it's likely because you woke up in the middle of deep sleep. This is the body repair phase, where tissues regenerate, muscles and bones rebuild, and the immune system strengthens. This is also when your mind gets some TLC, as the brain uses this time to commit important ideas to long-term memory and to rest and recharge for the next day. In fact, most of the major repercussions of sleep deprivation that we talked about earlier occur from not getting enough of *this* type of sleep. The longest stretches of deep sleep occur at the beginning of the night to ensure this healing happens, decreasing in later cycles as it becomes more and more complete.[17] For example, you might spend sixty minutes in deep sleep during your first cycle, followed by only forty minutes in the next. In fact, deep sleep can actually disappear altogether in the final cycles of your sleep session if all the necessary repairs are done.[18]

The final stage is REM sleep, called rapid eye movement because . . . well, your eyes start moving rapidly behind their lids. We have our most vivid dreams during this phase, but to make sure you don't act out the weird shit you're thinking, your brain actually *paralyzes* your limbs! Since this is the final stage before the end of a cycle, and your body is preparing to wake up briefly, your heart rate will increase, and your breathing will quicken.[19] This is a quick phase that typically lasts around ten minutes, though it's believed that REM sleep increases throughout the night as deep sleep decreases. If you regularly dream, that could be a good sign that REM has been extended because you're getting enough deep sleep.[20] REM sleep, in combination with deep sleep, refreshes the brain and improves memory storage, learning abilities, and mood.[21] After REM, you wake quickly, then it's back to the beginning of the cycle. The end?

Not quite. Understanding the sleep cycle is important, but no discussion of sleep is complete without bringing up the almighty circadian rhythm, which is the body's twenty-four-hour clock. You observe patterns every day with when you're hungry, sleepy, energized, focused, hell, even with when you need to poop. All of those behaviors are tied in with the circadian rhythm, and the better regulated it is, the more predictable the timing of those specific behaviors will be. Two parts of the regulation equation are the external cues of daylight and temperature.

Daylight is a critical trigger in regard to sleep. Shortly after the sun sets, our bodies know to start producing melatonin, which is the hormone that brings about the urge to sleep. That's different than our need for sleep, which is building up all day long. In fact, it starts accumulating as soon as we wake up. Think about one of those fundraiser temperature gauges—the need gradually increases as we use our brain and body throughout the day, and it hits the top of the gauge at night. When our sleep schedule is on point, the urge and the need neatly coincide, creating what's known as a sleep window, during which time it should be pretty easy to lie down and quickly drop into a sleep cycle.

For most adults, melatonin production begins naturally around 9:00 p.m. and starts triggering an urge to sleep. Production tapers off throughout the night and then halts as the sun rises. While melatonin is decreasing, cortisol production is increasing, peaking in the morning to help us wake. All of this is to say that, from a hormonal level, we're wired to go to bed and get up at specific times with relative ease. We just have to follow the instructions that we're getting from our bodies.

But if you're shaking your head right now and saying to yourself, *I'm not even tired until midnight!*, there's actually a scientific reason for that, too. During puberty, the adolescent body clock shifts by several hours, which causes the hormone production schedule to get out of whack until about age twenty.[22] This means your body may not be producing melatonin until around 11:00 p.m. *Sweet. Thanks, puberty!* Due to the late start, it then continues pumping out melatonin until well after the sun rises.[23] That's why, for some, going to bed before midnight or waking up early can be *really* tough during high school and college. Unfortunately, flexibility based on your sleep schedule doesn't really exist in high school, as classes tend to start at or before 8:00 a.m. In college, however, you have much greater control over your start time. The real trick is learning how to use that flexibility thoughtfully.

*"I slept a lot more in college than in high school. Being able to make my own schedule meant I was able to start classes later in the day (I hated having to get to high school by 8:00 a.m.), so I ended up getting a schedule that lined up a lot more with my natural sleeping schedule."*

—UNIVERSITY OF CALIFORNIA LOS ANGELES, RECENT GRAD

# ADJUSTED CIRCADIAN RHYTHM

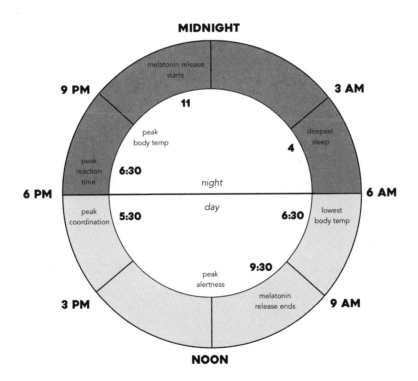

# Sleep Rules

It's time to talk about the "right" way to sleep. Feeling rested in the morning is possible regardless of when you go to bed, so long as you're working with your body. To avoid sleep deprivation and all of the unfortunate consequences it leads to, you have to control two things: the quantity and quality of your shut-eye.

## Quantity: Count Cycles Per Week, Not Hours Per Night

Eight hours is frequently cited as the average duration of a good night's sleep. Yet if you did the math as you were reading about sleep cycles—where the typical length is ninety minutes—eight hours is right in the middle of a cycle. Waking up with an alarm eight hours after your head hits the pillow could drop you right into the middle of NREM Stage 3. *Oh shit! You woke the bear!* To avoid this, measure sleep in cycles rather than hours. Five cycles of sleep yields about 7.5 hours, six cycles yields about 9 hours, and four cycles yields about 6 hours. Waking up at the end of a cycle will leave you feeling awake and refreshed, and five cycles per night is sufficient for most people's brains and bodies to take care of the required daily upkeep.

Five cycles every night is not always possible, and that's actually okay. According to elite sleep coach Nick Littlehales, each night is less important than each week.[24] This is a big deal because it allows for flexibility with daily quantity. Let's say you stay up late hanging out with friends or doing homework and can only squeeze in six hours of sleep. That shortage won't negatively affect you or contribute to overall sleep debt at all so long as you pay yourself back. You can do this by getting an extra cycle on another night or taking a full-cycle length nap during the day.

The goal: shoot for thirty-five cycles per week for an average of five cycles, or about 7.5 hours per night.[25] It's not the end of the world if you don't hit thirty-five each week, but do what you can to stay above twenty-eight. We're not fucking around! If you dip below twenty-eight cycles per week for two weeks straight, you will be in bad shape. This is the point where chronic sleep deprivation becomes a reality! A University of Pennsylvania study found that subjects who only got six hours of sleep every night for two weeks straight suffered impairment on par with missing two nights of sleep entirely.[26] Those scary and horrible repercussions we talked about before? You'll start to feel them if six hours becomes your norm. The scarier thing? You might not even be aware that you're suffering. According to the director of the UPenn study, the subjects only getting six hours stated they were slightly sleepy but didn't *think* their performance on the attention task they were required to regularly complete had decreased. In reality, their scores had plummeted.[27] Six hours might feel like enough rest, but according to the research, it's not enough to save you from damage.

## In Support of the Nap

Attention nap fans! Any speck of guilt you may have ever felt about sleeping during the day should now be destroyed. Why? Because naps can be a valid and valuable component of your weekly quantity calculations, as the almighty ninety-minute siesta can help you make up for missed cycles from the previous night or bank cycles for the busy days on the horizon. Naps aren't extra. They're secret weapons.

That said, timing is important to ensure that you drift off quickly, but don't interfere with your overnight sleep. Aim to start your nap between 1:00 and 3:00 p.m. Ever been hit with exhaustion in the afternoon? This slump actually happens for a reason. Your body temperature naturally drops during this time, triggering the release of melatonin, the same hormone that gets you sleepy at night. While this is the wrong time to focus on homework, this is the perfect time for a nap.

If you can't fit in a ninety-minute snooze, then a NASA-style power nap of between twenty and thirty minutes will still prove to be refreshing. Don't like short naps because you typically wake up wondering what day it is? Try adding coffee to the mix. That's right. Have some coffee, *then* go lie down. Some call it a coffee nap. Others, a nappuccino. But it works because it takes ten minutes after the first sip for the initial effects of caffeine to be felt, and maximum impact doesn't occur until the forty-five-minute mark, which times out with when you'd otherwise be struggling to rejoin the living. If you don't do caffeine, try washing your face or exposing yourself to bright light after waking up from any length nap; one study found those two methods to be on par with coffee in terms of regaining alertness.[28]

## Quality: Be Consistent

Even though your nightly quantity can vary, you've got to aim for consistency with when you go to bed and/or wake up. Studies show that dramatic changes in daily sleep habits wreak havoc on your circadian rhythm, meaning that your hormone production will be out of whack. Melatonin and cortisol won't assist you in falling asleep and waking up like they're supposed to, meaning you'll hit records with sheep counting at night and need buckets of coffee to pull yourself out of bed in the morning. One study of college students found that inconsistency with sleep schedule was almost as detrimental as not getting enough sleep per night, as the quality of the resulting sleep was so significantly impaired.[29]

The goal: keep sleep and wake times within the same two-hour window every day.[30] The easiest way to do this, and in turn keep your circadian rhythm on point, is to set an intention. Or, if we're just calling it like it is, give yourself a bedtime and wake time.

One option is to base your bedtime on when you typically start to feel sleepy and count about 7.5 hours forward to set your wake time. Bedtime, by the way, should be when your head hits the pillow and you turn out the lights, so you'll want to plan on calling it a night with friends or homework thirty minutes beforehand so that you can get ready. Another option is to set your wake time sixty minutes before your earliest class of the week. Sixty minutes will give you time to get ready and eat, plus, according to research, it takes that long to wake up fully. Then count backward 7.5 hours to find your bedtime. Of course, your class schedule changes every day, but try to keep your wake time roughly the same and use any extra minutes in the morning to finish schoolwork (use that morning focus window!) or squeeze in exercise. On a day when you're not going to get 7.5 hours of sleep, either because you're getting less, or God willing, more, try to change only your bedtime or wake time—not both. Regularity is key. In fact, to help out the ol' circadian rhythm, aim to get

*"My freshman-year roommate had a good system where she'd go to bed every night around 10:30 or 11:00 p.m. In hindsight, I should've done that, too. While 10:30 may seem a bit early to many people, the idea of a strict cutoff is valuable."*

—GEORGE WASHINGTON UNIVERSITY, SENIOR

four nights per week of identical sleep, meaning the same bedtime and wake time.[31]

*"My sleep habits are a disaster. Back in high school, I was usually in bed by 11:00 p.m. and asleep by midnight most days of the week since I had to wake up at 7:00 a.m. every morning. In college, the schedule is much more flexible but also much more out of control. For example, I've had quarters where I don't have class until 12:30 p.m., but I've also had times where I have a 9:30 a.m. class every day of the week. When you add the super late weekend nights onto that mess, there is just a huge amount of uncertainty about when you'll actually be in bed. I don't have a strict rhythm to my sleep schedule since it's changing day to day—which leads to some days where I'm super tired and other days where I'll be able to stay in bed as long as I want. It can't be the healthiest thing in the world."*

—NORTHWESTERN UNIVERSITY, JUNIOR

## Waking Up

If you can stick to those goals, you'll not only be able to exercise flexibility with your quantity a few nights each week, you'll simultaneously ensure quality sleep every night. When your circadian rhythm is in sync, you should effortlessly wake up feeling rested at the same time or within one cycle of your typical routine even on days when you don't set your alarm. But even when you are on point with consistency, getting out of bed can feel like torture some days. Here are four additional things you can do to help yourself get up and running in the morning:

- **Don't Press Snooze.** A tool for when you don't want to get up! Sounds great! Unfortunately, the time you spend in bed after pressing snooze is time wasted. As soon as you get jerked awake by an alarm, you're already out of a sleep cycle. Lying back down for fifteen minutes isn't going to leave you feeling more rested. It'll just leave you with less time to get ready. Only

# BEDTIME BASED ON CLASS TIME

| get ready | 10:00 p.m. | 10:30 p.m. | 11:00 p.m. | 11:30 p.m. | 12:00 p.m. | 12:30 p.m. | 1:00 p.m. | 1:30 p.m. |
| --- | --- | --- | --- | --- | --- | --- | --- | --- |
| lights-out | 10:15 p.m. | 10:45 p.m. | 11:15 p.m. | 11:45 p.m. | 12:15 p.m. | 12:45 p.m. | 1:15 p.m. | 1:45 p.m. |
| asleep by | 10:30 p.m. | 11:00 p.m. | 11:30 p.m. | 12:00 a.m. | 12:30 a.m. | 1:00 a.m. | 1:30 a.m. | 2:00 a.m. |

color coding below is based on the ideal wake up time for a first class that starts at:

| | 8 a.m. class | | 9 a.m. class | | | 10 a.m. class | | |
| --- | --- | --- | --- | --- | --- | --- | --- | --- |
| 4 cycles ~6 hrs | 4:30 a.m. | 5:00 a.m. | 5:30 a.m. | 6:00 a.m. | 6:30 a.m. | 7:00 a.m. | 7:30 a.m. | 8:00 a.m. |
| 5 cycles ~7.5 hrs | 6:00 a.m. | 6:30 a.m. | 7:00 a.m. | 7:30 a.m. | 8:00 a.m. | 8:30 a.m. | 9:00 a.m. | 10:00 a.m. |
| 6 cycles ~9 hrs | 7:30 a.m. | 8:00 a.m. | 8:30 a.m. | 9:00 a.m. | 9:30 a.m. | 10:00 a.m. | 10:30 a.m. | 11:00 a.m. |

snooze if you have time to lie down for another thirty or ninety minutes; otherwise, get your ass out of bed. Then . . .

- **Get Some Daylight.** Daylight helps your body produce serotonin, which is a hormone that enables you to feel calm, awake, and happy. You might consider sleeping with the curtains open so that the morning sun can aid in your wake-up efforts. Another option is using a sunrise alarm clock. These work by gradually emitting light, which allows your body to rise naturally. If all else fails, go outside. Until then . . .

- **Don't Check Your Tech.** Even if you're dying to know what you missed while sleeping, receiving texts, emails, and alerts is proven to induce stress. Keep in mind that your cortisol levels are already high when you wake up, so give your body a little time to recover before you check in on the world through your phone and jack them up even further.[32] Maybe while you're waiting, you can . . .

- **Move.** Stretch, do five push-ups, or take a walk to the bathroom. It doesn't matter what you do, moving helps your body temperature rise, which promotes feelings of alertness.

**But First, Water.** A glass of water to start the day is an excellent idea for more than its ability to help you battle dry mouth and bad breath. The solution to your morning fog may be as close as your water bottle. Here are two reasons to drink twelve ounces before you get going:

- **Water Will Energize You.** Well, frankly, the flip side is more accurate. Sleep is dehydrating, and not having the right amount of water in your system zaps your energy. When your body is low on fluids, your blood pressure drops, your heart rate quickens, and blood flow to your brain slows down.[33] All of this means that it will take more energy than usual to move blood, and therefore oxygen, to your cells, organs, and muscles, hence the drained energy. Dehydration can also be the root cause of feeling miserable during a morning (or any) workout. Your lungs and muscles are both about 80 percent water, and both go into emergency conservation mode when fluid levels are low, meaning they don't operate as intended. By having enough water in your system from the get-go, you allow your body to properly regulate energy usage, meaning you won't get hit with fatigue unexpectedly.
- **It'll Also Help You Focus.** Your brain is about 75 percent water, and when you're dehydrated, it panics. After all, it's got a shit ton of important jobs to do, such as controlling your thoughts, movements, and *vital organs*! So when it's having a freak-out, one of the first things to go is your focus and cognition, which only contributes to the haze that you may find yourself in after waking. For that reason, water first thing in the morning can be more powerful than coffee (which only further dehydrates you) at helping you fully join the living.

## Tracking Your Sleep

Technology can be a powerful ally in your quest to regularly get a solid quantity of good-quality sleep. Hundreds of thousands of people (myself and Jill included) swear by the app Sleep Cycle, which is an alarm clock . . . but better. Rather than setting a specific time you want to wake up, you set a window, say 7:15 a.m. to

7:45 a.m. The app uses the microphone in your phone to analyze your breathing as you sleep, then only sounds the alarm for you to wake once your breathing quickens, which is an indication that you're nearing the end of a sleep cycle.

Sleep Cycle not only tracks the amount of sleep you're getting per night but also produces a graph that summarizes how much time was spent in each stage (light sleep versus deep sleep) so that you have a better sense of your sleep quality. Additionally, it records the time at which you went to bed and woke up each day so that you can keep tabs on your consistency. Using this app or others like it can provide much-needed accountability where sleep is concerned.

---

**Symptoms of Chronic Sleep Deprivation.** Even without keeping tabs on hours of nightly sleep to make sure you're on track, you'll be able to tell if you're chronically sleep deprived based on how you're feeling and acting. Here is a list of common symptoms:[34,35]

- Excessive daytime sleepiness
- Difficulty falling or staying asleep (unfair, right!?)
- Abnormal movements or behaviors during sleep
- Constant sour mood or regular mood swings
- Poor memory and concentration
- Frequent fights with sickness and infection
- Hallucinations
- Body aches and pain
- Reduced sex drive

---

## Sleep Roadblocks

Getting enough sleep should be the easiest thing we can do for our health. It doesn't hurt like a hard workout, and it doesn't suck like passing on ice cream when you really want it. Literally, all you have to do is lie down in the most comfortable place you have access to and close your eyes, which sounds really easy to do. But it's not. Even with a clear understanding of both the downsides of not getting enough shut-eye and what's required to get a sufficient amount, there will be obstacles you'll need to overcome in your quest to become a sleep machine.

*"The freedoms that come with adulthood paired with the excitement of new peers and surroundings led to many sleepless nights in college. Even nights dedicated to studying became all-nighters as there are no parents to insist you close the books and turn out the lights."*

—THE NEW SCHOOL, RECENT GRAD

## People

It's common for sleep to lose in the battle against socializing. Particularly during freshman year, when everything is new and exciting and you're trying to make friends, hanging out often takes priority over sticking to a self-imposed bedtime. The simple advice is to look at those late nights as exceptions and not the rule. Think about nights of little sleep like junk food—let yourself stray from the "rules" when you're feeling like it, but hold yourself accountable. Don't feel guilty about staying up with friends a few nights each week, just make up for the time lost with extended sleep or naps on other days. One thing you definitely should try to avoid, however, is offering your room up as the place to hang out. As the host, you lose the freedom to bail and go to sleep when you're ready. Try to room with someone who is on the same page with that idea and also has similar sleep habits to your own.

*"FOMO (fear of missing out) is real, especially freshman year. I always felt that if I went to bed early, the most fun or exciting thing to happen all year would happen that night. Spoiler: it never did. Later in college, I started going to bed earlier, and guess what? I was so much happier and healthier in every way. And I could still spend time with my friends! The only things I missed out on were some movies that I didn't really want to see anyway, or games that we had already played a million times, or parties that got old real fast."*

—STANFORD UNIVERSITY, RECENT GRAD

## Work

If you don't manage your time well throughout the day, you may find yourself overwhelmed with the amount of work you still have left to do at night. We talked about some ways to deal with this overload and the stress that accompanies it in the last chapter, but what we *didn't* suggest was pulling an all-nighter to get caught up.

Twenty percent of college students pull an all-nighter on a weeknight at least once a month.[36] The overnight push can be helpful if you're out of time and the only goal is just to finish, but don't go this route if you're hoping to do quality writing or study material that you really need to know. Here's why.

First off, your memory actually becomes less functional when you're sleep deprived. Information needs to be stored as long-term memory to be accessed later, like during a test. The first part of committing something to long-term memory is acquisition—learning the material. Of course, this happens when you're awake. But information isn't stored without consolidation (the brain filing away the information as a memory) and this can't happen until you're asleep. Without adequate sleep, you might recognize an idea the next day but stand little chance of being able to recall it accurately.

Secondly, if you're staying up late to tackle a beastly paper or finish a project, it might not feel like your time was totally wasted, but it'll seem like you were. Sleep deprivation disrupts communication between brain cells, which is what causes impairment and makes you feel like you're in a fog. After seventeen to nineteen hours awake, your judgment, motor functions, and cognition are on par with someone with a BAC of .05. Stay up past twenty-eight hours, and that number climbs to .10.[37] Being acutely sleep deprived is like being drunk *and* extremely tired. Not a recipe for success.

What else could go wrong? Well, actually, a lot. As you push your sleep limits further and further, you're likely to experience confusion, memory loss, hallucinations, and distortions in time and personal perception, all eventually leading to acute psychosis.[38] You may fall asleep without warning, involuntarily collapsing into what is known as a "microsleep." Clearly, jumping onto the all-nighter train allows the consequences of procrastination to go far beyond added stress.

*"I only have one scar on my body—a two-inch, curvy guy on my right ankle. I got it my junior year when I pulled three all-nighters in a row and then fell asleep while riding my bike to my 8:00 a.m. class. I made it to the lab on time, but the instructor told me to go home because she didn't want me getting blood on the lab equipment."*

—UNIVERSITY OF SOUTHERN CALIFORNIA, RECENT GRAD

## Caffeine

More than 90 percent of college students consume caffeine, with coffee being the primary source, followed closely by tea, soda, and energy drinks.[39] Unsurprisingly, the most common reason to suck it back is to feel awake, and this wonder drug is effective because it actually tricks your body into thinking that you don't *need* sleep. Remember adenosine? The substance that accumulates all day, attaches to adenosine receptors, and then ultimately causes you to crave sleep? Scientists have seen that caffeine works by hip checking adenosine out of the way so that it can latch on to the adenosine receptors instead, thereby blocking feelings of sleepiness.[40] The one thing to keep in mind, however, is that the need is still very much there—caffeine is just tricking your body into not experiencing it. If you're curious about the ideal time to drink coffee, it's somewhere between 10:00 a.m. and noon,

*"I pull an all-nighter at least once a week. This really sucks the day after since I inevitably crash without meaning to or fall asleep during a lecture, but if I have a deadline, it means I do not sleep. This is common among my peers."*

—HARVARD UNIVERSITY, JUNIOR

after the morning cortisol spike has diminished and the need for sleep has started to accumulate slowly. But frankly, powering yourself with coffee anytime before 4:00 p.m. is fine. That time cutoff is based on a 2013 study, which showed that coffee can have disruptive effects on your shut-eye even six hours after it is consumed.[41] So try to consume caffeine during the first two-thirds of your day, and be sure to take in less than the recommended daily limit of 400 mg, which equates to about two energy drinks, four cups of coffee, or a whopping thirteen cups of tea.

**Tips for Pulling an All-Nighter.** As much as I'd love to convince you that pulling an all-nighter is stupid, I've been guilty of doing it many times. It almost always happened when I'd procrastinated too long and left myself no other option to meet a deadline. If you find yourself stuck in a similar situation, there are some ways you can reduce the amount of suffering you'll endure both during and afterward. Here are four policies to guide your overnight experience:

- **Space Out Coffee and Drink Water.** Don't exceed two cups of coffee during your overnight push. Sip it slowly with a snack in hand, and push water the rest of the time. Being hydrated will help you concentrate, and managing your caffeine intake will prevent you from getting jittery.
- **Skip Junk Foods.** Instead of eating exactly the garbage that you're craving, opt for small protein-heavy snacks throughout the night to prevent crashing—nuts, beef jerky, or full-fat yogurt are all portable choices. As we talked about in the last chapter, junk foods increase cortisol production, which will only add to the stress you're already putting on your body by being awake in the middle of the night.
- **Move.** Follow the ninety minutes on, twenty minutes off suggested work cycle from the last chapter, but specifically use the breaks to move around. Do some jumping jacks, push-ups, and squats, or go for a walk around your building. This will give your eyes a break from the computer screen while also getting your body temperature up, which will help you stay awake.
- **Sleep a Little!** Try for a full-cycle nap in the middle of your push if you can manage. If you don't have time for that, then shoot for a twenty- to thirty-minute power nap. Some rest is better than none.

It's equally important to take care of yourself the next day. Obviously, don't drive because you're basically drunk, but also drink plenty of water, don't overdo it with caffeine, take one ninety-minute nap, eat healthy meals, and exercise a little if you can. Then sleep hard. For a while.

## Booze

If you tend to get tired when you drink, then you might be under the impression that alcohol is good for sleep. While it will help you drift off quickly, booze has a strong negative impact on sleep quality, as it is specifically linked to a reduction in REM sleep. This means that the later cycles in your night, where deep sleep is reduced and replaced by more REM sleep, will be choppy and less restful.[42] This relationship works the other way as well; research has shown that those who get less sleep are more likely to have a negative relationship with alcohol.[43]

## Study Drugs

Studies have found that about a quarter of college students have used or regularly use study drugs, like Adderall or Ritalin, although less than 10 percent report having been prescribed them by a doctor.[44] Called "study drugs" due to the promise of improved focus and concentration, they're appealing because they seemingly make it possible to tackle challenging assignments and take on all-night pushes in preparation for exams. The downsides, however, are multiple.

First, these drugs mess with your sleep, which shouldn't be surprising not only because we're talking about them in this chapter, but also because they're considered stimulants. Usage impairs the circadian rhythm and sleep cycle, impacting both the quality and duration of rest when your body is ready for it. People wake up tired, compelled to take another pill or rely on caffeine to make it through the day, and those behaviors in turn compromise sleep for the next night. It can turn into a vicious cycle pretty quickly, particularly because both Ritalin and Adderall are Schedule II controlled substances, meaning that the risk of addiction or potential for abuse is high. For context, fentanyl, methadone, oxycodone, morphine, and opium are also on that list.

Now for the other concerns. When combined with alcohol, study drugs dull the symptoms of intoxication and can lead one to consume booze in extreme excess accidentally, potentially climbing to lethal levels. What's more, Adderall, in particular, is associated with an increased risk of depression and anxiety because it lowers dopamine production over time.[45] While these drugs might solve a short-term problem of keeping you alert enough to do your work when feeling overwhelmed, the repercussions of use will ultimately sabotage your overall physical and mental health. Stick with the suggestions outlined in the stress chapter when the pressure of work is mounting. These drugs aren't the answer.

## Technology

The blue background lights on our electronics hinder the production of melatonin.[46] Throw your phone and laptop on night mode so that you're staring into red-tinted light instead of blue. Warm, or red, tones don't inhibit melatonin production like cool tones do. In fact, studies show that red light actually increases melatonin production.[47] If you're willing to put down your devices but want to keep reading or doing homework up until you go to bed, invest in a warm-tone reading lamp. Check out Amazon for reading lights that can switch between warm/red and cool/ blue, so you can use them both during the day and at night.

## The Elements

When you're living in a dorm, you're at the mercy of others in regard to your exposure to light, noise, and heat, all of which can impact your ability to fall asleep. Here are four ways to regain control:

- **Light:** Bright light inhibits melatonin production, so if you want to sleep, you need to block it out. Light from the hallway can flood in under your door, so throw a blanket down to cover the crack, or try an eye mask—both are less suffocating than covering your head with a pillow.
- **Noise:** We're especially bothered by noise during the first two stages of a sleep cycle, which means anything loud or unpleasant can either prevent us from falling asleep or jerk us out of our place in a cycle altogether. To cut down on the sounds of your upstairs neighbor's late-night EDM parties, download a free white noise app on your phone and play it as you drift off. If that's not enough to shut the world out, buy some earplugs.
- **Heat:** In addition to melatonin, your body temperature is part of the grand sleep equation. When your body temperature is on the rise, you feel alert and awake. When it's on the decline, you feel sleepy. Internal temperature

regulation is tied to your circadian rhythm and production of melatonin,[48] but the outside environment also impacts how warm or cold you feel, and unfortunately, you won't typically have control over the temperature in your dorm room. If you're too hot, give your body some help by having a fan pointed at your bed. Additionally, if you're someone who tends to "run warm," avoid working out within two to three hours of when you plan to hit the sack. Exercise raises your core temperature, which makes you feel awake. Too cold? Get flannel sheets and wear warm clothes to bed.

- **Comfort:** Or lack thereof. Unless you're already in an off-campus apartment or live in your sorority or fraternity house, chances are good that you are sleeping on the lousy mattress that came with your dorm room. While these mattresses don't make the ideal base for the perfect sleep fortress, there are little things you can do to improve your comfort. First, get a foam or down mattress topper, depending on your firm/soft preference. This will also serve as a mattress protector (protecting you *from your mattress*). Second, get yourself some nice sheets. Ideally, hypoallergenic ones. To explain the reason for that, let's talk about dust mites for a moment. Dust mites are gross little microorganisms that like to make their home in carpets, curtains, mattresses, and bedding. They live off dust, yes, but they also eat skin flakes. Your skin flakes. *Eww.* You can't see dust mites, and you won't be allergic to the actual dust mite itself, but many people are allergic to dust mite secretions because they dry out and quickly become airborne. Yup, you heard me right. *Dust mite doodies, in the air. Dust mite doodies, everywhere.* Dust mites love college dorms, and while they aren't going to kill you or even make you sick, the idea of having them around is pretty gross, and an allergic reaction to them (sneezing, watery eyes, runny nose, congestion, trouble breathing) can make it really hard to sleep well.[49] To prevent dust mites from taking poops in your bed, you'll want to get hypoallergenic bedding. The tight weave of this bedding makes it impossible for dust mites to settle in, which is a win for you. Bedding, by the way, refers to the whole shebang: mattress pad, sheets, pillows, blankets. If you've already purchased this stuff but are still sneezing up a storm, no worries—keep your sheets and buy an air purifier instead.

## Rest Assured

Food and exercise are sexy areas of health. The ones that get the most attention. In 2020, the top twenty fitness influencers on Instagram had over one hundred million followers combined. The fact that the personalities behind these profiles are shredded and gorgeous has likely only furthered the belief that nutrition and movement are paramount in the effort to look like a well-styled bronzed god. We're eager to set goals for what we eat and how often we work out because we're programmed to believe that health is all about physical appearance.

But what about sleep?! Where are the shirtless influencers that want to commit to posting about their nightly bedtime routine? After all, sleep trickles down to every other area of our health. It gives us energy for exercise. It controls our appetites and impulses with alcohol. It regulates our circadian rhythm, which is what dictates the predictability of our focus windows. Sleep makes us feel great. Sleep allows us to kick ass. Sleep might not get the most coverage, but it shouldn't be overlooked in your efforts to look better, feel better, and do better. Be ready for the unique sleep challenges that will stand in your way once you get on campus, and do your best to prioritize rest despite the popular notion that less shut-eye is somehow a show of strength. If you're looking for a quick fix when it comes to your health, *this is it*. Get enough sleep, and the other areas will fall into place with much greater ease.

## For When You Forget

Because socializing, work, and streaming can feel like good reasons to push past your bedtime over and over again. When you come to the realization that you're sick of being a grumpy, red-eyed mess, start here:

- **Set a Bedtime.** Count backward 7.5 hours (five cycles) from the wake time you'd like to hit. Your wake time should ideally be sixty minutes before your first class, as this will give your mind a chance to become fully alert.

Getting up in the morning is easier when you base your bedtime on the desired number of sleep cycles (one cycle is about ninety minutes) rather than an arbitrary hour count, as our bodies automatically wake up at the end of a cycle anyway.

- **Consistency is Key.** Shoot for four identical days of sleep per week by going to bed and waking up at about the same time. Outside of those four days, try to keep all bedtimes within the same two-hour window. The same goes for wake times. This will help keep your circadian rhythm regulated, which will make falling asleep and waking up easier in general.

- **Strategize to Hit a Weekly Goal.** There is room for flexibility when it comes to sleep, as the ideal quantity is actually thirty-five cycles *per week*. Although this breaks down to a nightly average of five cycles or 7.5 hours, those cycles can be reallocated. A six-hour night can be balanced out by a nine-hour night or a long daytime nap. Thirty-five cycles may not be possible every week, but attempt to stay above twenty-eight, as regularly only getting four cycles (or six hours) per night puts you in the danger zone for chronic sleep deprivation.

Try to remember:

- **Control What You Can.** Get a noise machine, sleep mask, fan, mattress pad, hypoallergenic sheets, and whatever else you need to create a kick-ass sleep environment. One so cozy and relaxing that the idea of being anywhere else after midnight is entirely unappealing.

- **Know the Warning Signs of Chronic Sleep Deprivation.** If you're not getting enough sleep, it'll impact other areas of your life. Keep an eye on your mood, your grades, and your body. If things are taking a nosedive and you can't understand why (*but I'm studying so hard that I'm pulling regular all-nighters!*), there's a good chance that lack of sleep is to blame. Give yourself permission to go to bed. You're the motherfucking boss now.

# CHAPTER 7
# TRIAL AND ERROR

### JILL

**One morning recently, Dave and I woke up before sunrise to go for a run.** He typically takes a while to warm up to the world in the early hours, requiring at least two cups of coffee before he's ready to communicate with full sentences. Still, his energy was particularly dark on this day. I'm pretty sure he muttered, "I hate everything," as he slowly tied his shoes. We made it halfway through our regular loop in silence before he exclaimed matter-of-factly, "I feel terrible." It wasn't a plea for help; there was no urgency in his voice. Instead, he was genuinely surprised. Like his body had been keeping secrets and revealed to him all at once its symptoms of displeasure.

"Well . . . let's talk about it."

We started down the checklist of potential culprits. He'd been eating okay recently, limiting his ice cream destruction to weekends. He was relatively hydrated and had been exercising a decent amount each week. There was stress at work, but not so much where he was in danger of lighting his boss's office on fire.

"When was the last time you got a good night of sleep?"

His silence lasted a while, only disturbed by the sounds of our breathing and running shoes on pavement, before reluctantly admitting the truth—he couldn't remember. For weeks, maybe even months, Dave had been getting less than six hours of sleep each night, staying up late so he could unwind. While that time was intended to bring levity to days that were mostly spent at work, the consequence was clear. He was chronically sleep deprived.

In the process of working on this project, we've both become more convinced than ever that good health is fluid. There's not a switch you can flip and be forever changed. Your current state is just a reflection of the recent choices you've made. Maybe you'll stay up all night playing video games only to wake up with your arm around a box of pizza. Maybe you'll avoid the gym for a solid month. Maybe you'll drink for seven days straight. Maybe you'll fall behind on your work and get to a point where you feel nauseous just thinking about how much you have to do. Maybe you'll just eat too many gross snacks. The reality is that you are forced to make countless decisions *every single day* that impact your health. You won't always make the best ones, and you won't always course-correct quickly when you fall out of your good routines. The real key to being healthy? Finding your way back to it over and over again by recognizing when you're off track, and then deliberately making a plan to get to where you want to be.

The recipe for overall good health is trial and error. It always begins with the personal acknowledgment of feeling like shit, coupled with a desire to do better that is stronger than the temptation to make excuses and let yourself off the hook. In this chapter, we will walk you through everything from identifying the problem (which we'll call the pretrial), to designing and testing solutions (trial), to moving forward when you get off track *yet again* (error). Dave and I have spent years and years putting *work* into being healthy because that's what it requires. We don't live in a perpetual state of perfect. In fact, we regularly fail to take care of ourselves like we know we should. But we have succeeded in our ability to start over, and those experiences have filled us with the confidence to know that it's *always* possible to fix what feels broken. All you have to do is begin.

## Pretrial: Where Are You At?

Just as crap fuel and insufficient maintenance will compromise even the nicest car, those same things will also make your body feel terrible. The way your body functions is dependent on what you're putting into it and how you're taking care of it. That's why, when you come to the realization that your body and/or mind is in a bad place, it's important to pay attention to your current situation with food, booze, exercise, stress, and sleep. When you slide with regularity in any one of those areas, you threaten to trigger the creation of inflammation. While inflammation is usually the first step in your immune system's effort to help you feel better, too much of it can also be what causes you to feel like trash.

Acute versus chronic. Quick to pass versus incessant and draining. You've heard these terms before in regard to stress and sleep deprivation, but they're also used to categorize inflammation. Acute inflammation is the good kind. It's what you see when you cut your finger, sprain your ankle, stub your toe, or have a sore throat. Localized redness and swelling are the way your body drops a road flare, communicating the message "attention needed here!" At this point, cytokines, the infection-fighting warriors we talked about in the sleep chapter, flock to the site, work their magic, and fix the problem. When healing is well on its way, the inflammation dissipates.

However, it doesn't always present itself externally and fade quickly. Introducing chronic inflammation! The bad kind. This is the result of an injury to the body that can't be promptly healed because the source of the issue is persistent. This type of inflammation is linked to a whole host of diseases, but the basic symptoms of it— body pain, fatigue, moodiness, weight gain, and gastrointestinal discomfort—are unpleasant enough all on their own.[1] And what, you ask, causes this type of everlasting inflammation? Repeated behaviors that don't serve the body, like a diet packed with sugar and processed food, inadequate or inconsistent sleep, an overload of stress, or regular use of alcohol or other drugs.[2] And though lack of exercise doesn't cause chronic inflammation, incorporating movement is cited as one of the best ways to prevent it. This is why you need to consider the areas we discussed in this book when you feel lousy. "I feel terrible" can be fixed, but it will only happen once you're willing to honestly consider the actions that got you there in the first place. And that part isn't always easy.

## Your Honor Code

I remember being thrilled when the Screen Time app came out on the iPhone. I feel like I'm more detached from my phone than many people and couldn't wait to review my results at the end of the first week. Those numbers were going to give me a pathetic excuse to feel good about myself! When the alert came up on Sunday morning, I opened the app and studied the data. *Four hours and thirty-five minutes. Not bad!* Until I noticed that number was my average per day. *How in the hell is that possible? Two hours on Instagram? Son of a bitch!* The information was startling. *Welp, not looking at that anymore.* But I didn't mean Instagram. I was referring to the Screen Time app.

This type of behavior is known as "information aversion," and it's common among everyone, especially where our health is concerned. People actually have a tendency to avoid the truth if we believe it's going to cause us stress or anxiety.[3] When we encounter a setback, we tend to judge ourselves, and that judgment doesn't typically feel good. It's natural to want to avoid that pain and ignore underlying problems altogether. However, that doesn't usually result in problems solved. If you feel like garbage, the first step toward finding a fix is to *accept it*. Admit the truth. It'll feel good to start surging (or slothing) toward a solution. And it's better than wallowing away in a stagnant, sleep-deprived, stress-filled, sugar shitstorm of sadness.

## Time Check

Time is the most valuable currency we have when it comes to well-being. It's required to move the dial on the "give-a-shit-about-health-o-meter," because it takes time to exercise, to meal prep, to get work done, and to sleep. If you feel stretched thin trying to stay on top of your health, take a moment to honestly identify how you're spending time. Then use that information to earn some of it back.

Technology is a universal time suck. A 2014 study found that on an average day, college students spend 95 minutes texting, 65 minutes on social media, 57 minutes sending emails, 35 minutes surfing the internet, and 33 minutes making calls.[4] Surely those numbers have only risen since then, considering apps and social media platforms are continuously introduced. That's also not counting streaming, though a 2018 Nielsen Media Research report found that the average person spends nearly six hours each day watching video content across all platforms.[5] In total, college women in one study reported spending an average of 600 minutes on their phones each day.

In contrast, men reported spending about 460 minutes.[6] Just so we're clear, that's ten *hours* and almost eight *hours*, respectively. I'm not even sure how that's possible, though given how shocked I was by my own device usage, I'm inclined to believe those numbers.

Research has found that, among college students, device dependence is mostly born out of a desire to connect with others. However, time spent on social media, in particular, was found to be associated with cell phone addiction,[7] which, ironically, is linked to feelings of isolation and loneliness.[8] We're using our phones to socialize but are ultimately left feeling sad and alone. *Womp womp.* Additionally, streaming content has been found to steal time away from schoolwork for students specifically.[9] So it seems that all of the time we're spending in front of screens is not only taking time away from the things we could be doing for our health, it's contributing to added stress, which only further pushes us away from where we want to be.

### *Excuses, Excuses*

We use excuses to let ourselves off the hook—they allow us to give in to temptations without feeling guilty. *I'm tired. I feel sick. I've had an awful day.* Excuses help us protect ourselves from the sting of failure when we believe it's inevitable.[10] Maybe you did have a shitty day. Perhaps you are exhausted. You might need sleep more than you need to work out. But maybe you're just feeling unmotivated and would rather watch TV than sweat, so you're coming up with reasons that seem more legitimate than "I don't feel like it" to avoid being disappointed with yourself later?

Again, the first part of getting around this is being honest with yourself. Drift from your path, but don't fabricate the reason it happened. If you don't feel like doing something, that's fine! Just don't kid yourself about what's going on. The problem with excuse-making is that the more we do it, the easier it becomes. You start to convince yourself that there's real legitimacy in your excuses. Studies show that missing a day here or there doesn't seriously impair our ability to stick with good routines,[11] but problems arise when we allow ourselves to check out too often. Do this, and you become *that* person. The type of person who says one thing and does another. Someone who always has a reason they *can't* rather than a fiery determination to "I can" the shit out of everything. Someone who doesn't raise the bar for themselves. Don't let yourself be *that* person. If you don't want to do something, *own it*. Don't let excuses make you their bitch. If you think there might actually be some truth at the root of your excuses, then go back to the beginning and ask yourself *why*. Are you tired? *Why?* You feel sick? *Why?* Assess the situation, find the underlying problem, and then *fix it* so that you can stop the bullshit train in its tracks.

Whether it's avoidance or excuses, your health will suffer if you aren't honest with yourself. So take a deep breath in, release a little ego on the way out, and then objectively and truthfully analyze your recent behavior. It's the only way to fully understand *why* you're feeling the way you feel.

## Breaking It Down

Being honest with yourself is essential to identifying missteps with your health, but admitting to your shortcomings with exercise isn't enough. It can be easy to recognize macroproblems with different areas of health. The harder task is identifying the multitude of seemingly insignificant microbehaviors that are causing them. Sometimes they're not even in the same area. For example, let's say you're having a tough time sticking to your morning workout. Unfortunately, it's the only time you have during the day to exercise, so you've got to make it work. Perhaps wolfing down that big bowl of ice cream after dinner every night is actually the problem. The sugar could be disrupting your sleep, causing you to wake up tired and groggy rather than ready to get after it. Maybe you need to scrap the dessert at night to kick ass at the gym in the morning.

I can't presume to identify which microbehaviors are causing *your* macroproblems, but I can remind you that you now have a clear idea of what it looks like to be healthy with food, booze, exercise, stress, and sleep. You've got the cheat codes for making changes! Use that knowledge and work backward. Where are you drifting from what's considered healthy? Everyone's strengths, weaknesses, and vices are different. Some people have a lot of trouble committing to sleep, others can't seem to kick junk food. More still are terrible procrastinators who are always one step away from having a stress-related meltdown. My microstruggles seem to change constantly. However, the more you do this type of work, the easier it becomes to identify your issues. You may even start to see patterns with what caused you problems in the past. When it's time to check in with yourself, honestly peel back the layers of your behavioral onion and figure out which small decisions are causing your large problems. Once you've identified what needs attention, then you can go about fixing it.

## The Trial: Focus on Habits

Health is ruled by habits. The good ones we hold make it easier to stay on track, and the bad ones secretly sabotage us. Habits are more complex than you might think. In essence, habits are regularly repeated routine behaviors that happen without much attention and mental energy.[12] Which is simultaneously awesome and scary. Your brain loves habits, as they remove the effort from mundane actions, which in turn saves energy for challenging ones. Once a routine becomes a habit, you won't have to think about how to get it started or what it entails. I put on shoes every single day, and I literally have no idea how I tie them. I'm sure it involves a loop and swoop, but I couldn't tell you where because it's a habit. Same with brushing my teeth, driving to a familiar place, or watching rom-coms. Seriously. Sometimes I just find myself in front of the TV weeping into a bowl of chips, and I have no idea how I got there. Habits, man.

But we have more automatic processes programmed into our human brains than shoe tying and toothbrushing. Nearly 45 percent of our regular actions are habits, occurring at the same time and in the same place every single day,[13] which is pretty insane if you think about it; up to half of what the average human does while awake is a routine that unfolds without permission or effort. *I bet you never knew you were part robot.* However, the power of the habit, when harnessed, can change your life in the very best way. Once you understand how a habit works, you'll have the ability to add ones to your life that will make it easier or change any existing ones that aren't helping you out. Habits are the secret sauce that ass-kickers around the world use to kick ass on tasks without even thinking about them. They're also metaphorical power tools and concrete that you're going to use to fix your crumbling health foundation when needed.

## The Habit Blueprint

Habits have three specific components, which *New York Times* reporter and author Charles Duhigg discussed in his 2012 book, *The Power of Habit*: "First, there is a cue, a trigger that tells your brain to go into automatic mode and which habit to use. Then there is the routine, which can be physical or mental or emotional. Finally, there is a reward, which helps your brain figure out if this particular loop is worth remembering for the future. Over time, this loop becomes more and more automatic. The cue and reward become intertwined until a powerful sense of anticipation and craving emerges."[14] In essence, the cue is the start button, the routine is the behavior itself, and the reward is what you get or feel as a result of going through the motions. It may sound like a dance number for dog treats, but knowing the pieces that make up a habit can be used to deliberately guide your trial when it's time to test out solutions.

### *Routine*

While it may seem like we're going out of order here, a good first step is to identify the behavior that you want to make automatic. Think you can't exercise in the morning because you're overeating ice cream at night? Troubleshoot! Replace all of that ice cream eating with something that should theoretically contribute to your health and get you out the door in the morning. Maybe it's tea, perhaps it's a long shower, maybe you just need to get in bed earlier. Test some shit out. This is the trial phase, after all! Whatever your problem, script an easy-to-follow routine that aims to fix it or helps you avoid it, and be sure to establish specifics mindfully. The more you can plan, the better your chance of success.

### *Cue*

Next up is your habit's "on" button—the cue. The cue is what separates a random routine from an ingrained habit. All of your existing habits have cues, so if you want to introduce a new one in your life, it makes sense to determine ahead of time what exactly is going to trigger it. The cue will act as a reminder until your habit is formed, after which point it'll just operate as the subconscious trigger. According to James Clear, Habits Academy creator and author of *Atomic Habits*, there are five common habit cues:[15]

1. **Preceding Event.** Example: "After I take a shower, I make my to-do list for the day." Also known as anchoring, the idea is that you can use the completion of an existing habit to cue the beginning of a different one.

2. **Time.** Example: "Upon waking up in the morning, I brush my teeth." A specific or general time of day can be used to initiate your habit. According to Clear, this is the most common habit cue.

3. **Location.** Example: "As soon as I walk into the dining hall, I fill up my water bottle." You can use a change in an environment to prompt a habit.

4. **Emotional State.** Example: "When I'm bored, I check my phone." Clear believes the way we're feeling often jump-starts bad habits. What are your go-to behaviors when you're tired, stressed, sad, excited, angry, annoyed, or bored? If they aren't positively contributing to your life, work on replacing them with something else that would.

5. **People.** Example: "When I'm hanging out with friends who are all eating well, I also eat well." Research shows that the habits of those around you affect your behavior,[17] for both the better and worse. Spend your time with other ass-kickers, and you'll be continuously cued to kick ass.

*"I've found that when I'm surrounded by people who have good habits regarding food, exercise, and alcohol, I want to stick to good habits more."*
—DURHAM UNIVERSITY, SENIOR

## Reward

You're much more likely to maintain a habit if you're getting something desirable out of it. The reward is the final piece of the blueprint, but arguably the most crucial component to connect with. Rewards can be broken down into two separate categories, which I know already sounds like a really boring way to talk about a benefit, but stick with me; it's actually kind of important. Extrinsic rewards are tangible things you receive for completing a task. Food, money, gadgets, grades, praise. They are external incentives. Starting to exercise so that you can have ice cream after dinner is an excellent example of a habit that is attached to an extrinsic

**Willpower Isn't Your Problem.** If you've tried to make changes before and failed, then perhaps you believe that success isn't in the cards for you. That you're just weak-willed and incapable of sticking to your guns and meeting your goals. Think again. Willpower isn't a gift that some receive and others don't. It's a limited resource that drains quickly when tapped into, and facing temptation is like cutting the bottom off the barrel. A study at McGill University found that when students had to put *effort* into self-control in order to reach their goals, they became exhausted from exercising restraint. Ultimately, they were less likely to succeed as a result.[16] The key isn't self-control. That's hard for everyone. The key is effort. Particularly, figuring out how to reduce the effort required to make good choices.

One obvious way to minimize the need for self-control is to remove temptations wherever possible. Another is to design habits so that your good choices become automatic. If you want to really increase the chance that those habits will stick, focus on adopting routines that you find enjoyable. Determine which healthy foods you actually like eating. Exercise by doing something you look forward to at a time of day that doesn't feel like punishment. Give yourself breaks within work pushes so you don't feel like a prisoner when it's time to sit down and get started. Establish a bedtime or wake time routine that you look forward to in some way so it's easier to regulate your sleep schedule. If you specifically look to script routines that you know you will be excited about, the effort required to hold onto them will be much less.

reward. Even exercising so someone will tell you, "Hey . . . sweet abs," is another extrinsic reward. They're nice because they are effortless to create—*Pizza Friday if I have a good week!*—but unfortunately, studies show that the power of the prize wears off over time. The allure of tangible rewards becomes less and less powerful the more frequently you receive them. In his 2011 book about motivation, titled *Drive*, author Daniel Pink summarizes other problems that emerge when the emphasis is solely placed on extrinsic rewards: they promote short-term thinking, weaken performance, and reduce intrinsic motivation.[18] So how do you reward yourself in a way that will bring lasting satisfaction?

Intrinsic rewards are the golden ticket. You experience them when you are doing something you find inherently interesting that gives a sense of achievement upon completion. That feeling you get at the end of the day when you know you worked hard and did a good job? That's an intrinsic reward. They're like happiness bombs. *BOOM!* And not the type of happiness that flashes when someone gives you a compliment or hands you a beautiful bowl of ice cream. Rather, it's a joy that fills you up and makes you smile even when no one is there to see it. Intrinsic rewards can come in many shapes and sizes and be different for each person—some people get a kick out of tackling tasks that are challenging or displaying mastery of a complicated skill set, while others gravitate towards letting their curiosity run wild.[19] When you engage in a behavior simply because you know it'll satisfy your soul, the by-product can be as simple as forgetting about the things that are bothering you to as extreme as temporarily separating from your perceived identity and potentially transcending ego boundaries.[20] In other words, connecting to intrinsic rewards can really help you pull your head out of your ass and deeply grow as a human being. *Dope!* Habits are meant to be lifelong routines. Ones that will hopefully set you up to make great decisions with your health while removing the effort. So, if you're trying to pick up a habit for the long run, don't plan around a reward that will, at some point, feel unrewarding. It's better, instead, to identify the internal payoff that you experience after completing the routine. Dave and I work out because we know, without fail, we will always feel good physically and mentally once it's over. That assurance has come with time and experience. If you're new to trying something, there's nothing wrong with using extrinsic motivation to help you make healthy choices in the beginning. I can promise, however, that once you start taking care of yourself simply *because* it makes you feel good, you'll realize there's no greater reward.

**Intrinsic Motivation Triggers.** Looking to design habits that are guaranteed to make you feel good *inside*? According to theorists Thomas Malone and Mark Lepper, seven factors encourage intrinsic motivation and result in intrinsic rewards.[21] Four of them are particularly well suited to be the driving force behind habits that impact our physical and mental health:

- **Challenge.** Look for routines that will be difficult enough to challenge you, but not so difficult that they are frustrating. This way, you will feel a tremendous amount of pride when you complete them. This could include something physically challenging, such as doing push-ups every day, or mentally challenging, such as skipping dessert on weeknights.
- **Control.** Routines that help you gain control over your life and environment—cleaning your room, making a to-do list, or having a meal plan—may provide you with feelings of inner peace and confidence.
- **Competition.** Games or contests have a way of turning mundane or dreaded routines into an event, leaving you feeling excited and engaged. Those of you with an Apple Watch who are obsessed with closing your rings every day probably understand this best.
- **Cooperation.** Including someone else in your routine, such as deciding on a bedtime with your roommate and encouraging each other to stick to it at night, can be very effective. Not only will you have built-in accountability, but you'll also feel joy as a result of connecting over a shared challenge.

# Get Testing

As mentioned earlier in the book, I used to really struggle with making good choices at meals in college. Soft serve over a salad any day of the week. There are still days I'd rather eat a pile of carbs covered in cheese than vegetables. That said, I know how terrible my body feels when I eat like shit. I eventually decided to adjust my routine by adopting a super simple habit: I start with vegetables. When it's time to eat, they're the first thing I put on my plate. That's it. I only do this at lunch and at dinner. I'm pretty tough, but I'm not "vegetables for breakfast" tough. My cue is the preceding event of grabbing a plate, my routine is using veggies to cover half of it, and my reward is that I'm proud of myself for eating well. This habit has helped me strike a balance at most mealtimes without an ounce of effort, and it's contributed to the development of other good habits, like meal planning and food prep.

> **Small Changes, Big Payoffs.** It's entirely possible to read a book, watch a doc, or listen to a podcast with no intention other than to be entertained, only to finish feeling completely compelled to overhaul your entire life. All at once. Big mistake. Not only does a full-scale change end up requiring a fair amount of money, time, and effort, it doesn't usually stick. The key? Look to incorporate habits that are small in terms of time and effort required. Here's why:
>
> - **Easier to Start and Maintain:** Obviously, adding new behaviors to your daily routine will require an adjustment, but the less they demand, the more quickly they'll become comfortable. Anything comfortable will be easy to maintain, and after you maintain something long enough, the bar for what you consider normal in your life will adjust.
> - **Gain Confidence:** Successfully adding or changing a habit will contribute to your belief that change is possible. That *you* are capable of taking action and following through. There's no substitute for a positive experience when it comes to building confidence in yourself.
> - **Small Things Add Up:** Taking care of yourself is a big job comprised of small behaviors. The only way to keep tabs on the full range of your health is to spend time locking down individual habits. This can't be rushed, but the sum of your efforts, no matter how long it takes, will serve you for the rest of your life.

This is just one example of how using habits can help you right the ship when you're not where you want to be. Our intention with this book is to provide you with the tools to do an honest and knowledgeable assessment of your health. Your circumstances and wellness will change throughout college and for the rest of your life, but once you know what good health looks like, you'll always be able to determine where you're at and what you can do to course correct.

Building habits is a great way to take some of the work out of every single one of those restarts. Some of the habits you attempt will stick, and you'll never need to put effort into that area of your health again. Some will be forgotten almost immediately. Playing around with habit creation, however, is a worthy investment of time. It's a trial and error that will result in you continuously cultivating a relationship with your body and mind, which will gradually strengthen your health foundation.

| AREA | THE GREATEST COLLEGE HEALTH PRACTICES |
|---|---|
| FOOD | • Load up half your plate with vegetables before adding other foods.<br>• Replace mindless late-night snacking with gum, tea, or something healthy.<br>• Pack or plan for a quality snack in the middle of your day.<br>• Replace your afternoon sugar-filled caffeine fix with a decaf plain latte or coffee.<br>• Replace soda with sparkling water.<br>• Establish one or two healthy weekday breakfast go-to's.<br>• Replace dessert after lunch with fruit.<br>• Replace late-night weekend pizza with cereal or pretzels.<br>• Drink a full bottle of water before having seconds at any meal.<br>• Make a weekly menu and meal prep every Sunday. |
| BOOZE | • Set a drink limit for the night before you go out.<br>• Alternate between water and booze.<br>• Start the "morning after" with a sports drink or coconut water.<br>• Say no to shots altogether or limit yourself to one each time you go out.<br>• Make a deal with a friend to look out for each other. |
| EXERCISE | • Make a weekly workout plan on Sunday.<br>• Always plan for a Monday workout.<br>• Plan to work out with a friend once or twice each week.<br>• Wear workout clothes to class so that you can hit the gym when you're done.<br>• Schedule in a class once or twice a week to keep yourself motivated. |
| STRESS | • Before you check your phone while bored, take three super deep breaths.<br>• Keep a water bottle by your bed and take a few slugs as soon as you wake up.<br>• Plan out tomorrow before going to bed tonight.<br>• Start each day by taking care of yourself.<br>• Schedule in homework time and observe focus windows for maximum productivity.<br>• Write in a journal or talk to a friend when you're feeling overwhelmed. |
| SLEEP | • Set a bedtime/waketime routine and stick to it most nights.<br>• Stretch in bed instead of pressing snooze.<br>• Stop caffeine after 4 p.m.<br>• Brush your teeth before you check your phone in the morning. |

Being healthy is a practice that requires regular work, self-awareness, and real desire. We can't give you those things. What we can give is a habit road map to get you headed in the right direction and a pile of suggestions to keep you on track.

## Getting Ahead of Obstacles

Starting a new habit is exciting, and that alone will usually propel you forward for the first few weeks. However, truly sticking to good behaviors—especially those in areas where you commonly struggle—isn't easy. Scripting out your routine and picking a great cue with a reward that should resonate is an excellent start. Still, according to a study from 2009, it takes, on average, just over two months (sixty-six days) to cement a habit.[22]

Preparation alone won't save you from the temptation demons. Your resolve will be challenged at some point, and it's best to prepare for the inevitability of setbacks. Be honest with yourself about where you're expecting struggle so you can get ahead of it, and try to decrease your access to the things that you know will knock you off track. To do that, consider implementing any of these five strategies:

1. **Capitalize on Ease.** Make your good behaviors so convenient that more energy is required to avoid doing them than to follow through. For instance, wear your workout clothes to class, and you won't have to walk back to your room to change before heading to the gym. You'll save time, while also altogether avoiding the temptation of dropping into your bed and taking a nap instead.

   If you're trying to cut out a bad habit, the flip side of this approach is compelling as well. Leverage hassle. Make adjustments to your life so that your disruptive and destructive behaviors suddenly require a whole lot more effort.[23] Eating an entire bag of Cheetos is a much bigger time and energy suck if it requires the preliminary steps of putting on clothes and shoes and walking to the store, rather than just snatching the family-size bag you bought at Target out of a drawer in your room. Find ways to make positive microbehaviors quick and straightforward and negative ones time consuming and cumbersome.

2. **Plan Your Alternative.** When you're attempting to steer clear of something you typically crave, urges can feel unbelievably powerful. For any urges you find

yourself regularly struggling to overcome, formulate, ahead of time, the sub-sequent course of action that will direct you toward your desired outcome.[24] So, for example, if you're hit with the desire to have another drink, but you know that you've reached your limit, then you could avoid it with the help of a replacement, such as a glass of water, a distraction, like playing a game of pool, or a change of scenery—perhaps it's time to leave the party. Ultimately, it's about anticipating where you tend to have trouble and planning ahead. Be honest with yourself and play to your strengths when planning your alternative, because, for it to work, it must be compelling enough to help you move past your urge.

3. **Make Adjustments.** Even the best-laid health plans can go to shit when unex-pected obligations disrupt your regular schedule, which happens especially often in college. If you see a conflict between your habit and another event on the horizon, make it a priority to reschedule one or the other. For instance, if your parents are in town and you have plans to go out to dinner, move your eve-ning exercise routine to the morning just for the day. If a last-minute meeting comes up that derails your plan to go for a sixty-minute run in the afternoon, do a twenty-minute run or a quick strength circuit in your room instead. Don't let changes to your schedule become excuses. Your schedule will always be in flux, and you'll never achieve peak health if you continually let yourself off the hook because of it. Be flexible and make adjustments when necessary.

4. **Hold Yourself Accountable.** Feeling beholden to something or someone can be valuable when you're trying to stay on track. It doesn't work for everyone, but for the other people pleasers out there, accountability can be a powerful tool. Having others invested in your progress will help you stick to your plan,[25] so if you're trying to make a change, tell someone about it. Specifically, tell some-one who you know will follow up. Make it someone whom you don't want to disappoint. If you want to go a step further, surround yourself with friends who are busy testing out habits and kicking ass. Pass this book along to them when you're done so that you're all on the same page. It is possible to adopt the self-control cues of others if you're exposed to them enough.[26] That said, there are certain habits you may not want accountability buddies for. A 2014 study

showed that when the stakes of sacrificing a habit are high, something like "give up drinking," people bond through moral support. However, when the stakes are low, such as "don't eat sweets at night," it's incredibly easy, even fun, to fall into the partner-in-crime trap and make excuses with someone.[27]

The only thing you have to be careful about with this one is getting tricked into feeling like you've already achieved something by simply putting it out there. There is research that says discussing your goals with others and experiencing their praise can result in the same type of rush that you'd get from *actually* reaching the goal. In other words, simply *saying* you're going to do something will feel good enough that *actually* doing it won't be necessary.[28] The only way to figure out if this type of thinking applies to you is to try it. If you regularly vocalize goals and then don't reach them, keep your plan of action to yourself until you're almost at completion. You can hold yourself accountable by using an app to monitor your habit: record your workout, what you eat, how long you sleep, or how much water you drink. There are even apps that simply keep track of the number of days you've stuck to a habit. Technology can be a powerful ally in helping you maintain your habits, as being aware of your progress may lessen the temptation to quit.

*"One thing I wish I had started earlier is keeping track of daily sleep, exercise, nutrition, and how I felt. It would've been easy to do with some fitness/lifestyle app, and I think it would've been really powerful to see how those aspects of my life were working with or against each other, especially during freshman year as I was adjusting to college life."*
—UNIVERSITY OF CALIFORNIA, BERKELEY, SENIOR

5.  **Take a Break.** Assume burnout is inevitable and plan for breaks. It's essentially the rest day concept of exercise applied across the board. Employing this strategy means you won't have to make excuses to have some fun. Arrange for food indulgences, late nights, and days off from exercise so you don't feel deprived. A scheduled break from a habit feels special—it's something you'll look forward to, which means you'll enjoy it all the more when it arrives. The awesome side

effect is that these breaks will also prevent future impulsive deviations, meaning you're more likely to stick to your plan day in and day out. Just a tip—be sure you know the end date of your break.

## The Error: It's Not Failure

Even if you're an ass-kicking habit creator who never gives in to excuses, you're going to have numerous setbacks with your health in your life because you're human! We make mistakes. The idea of starting over implies failure, like the video game you couldn't beat and had to head back to the beginning of the level. Rather than feeling like a loser . . . again . . . and beginning another metaphorical walk of shame, look at these opportunities as what they are: a chance to try again. To start *fresh*. That means letting go of any feelings you may be attaching to your current situation and the decisions that led there. Guilt and shame may be powerful motivational tools in Catholic school, but they will only weigh you down in the long run. Drop that shit. Drop it right now. To make progress, you should remove every possible obstacle, especially the tendency to feel bad about yourself. You're going to be in this body for your whole life—it's about time you two became friends. When it's time to start up again, give yourself a clean slate.

As a college student, you experience multiple significant beginnings within a year—the start of the first semester, winter break, second semester, spring break, and summer break. A change in circumstance or schedule provides an excellent opportunity to make adjustments to your habits. Of course, you don't need a momentous occasion to shake things up. Monday is fine too. If you really need to make a change, the right moment should be the nearest one.

## Rethink

After the struggle bus has circled back for you and you've finally decided it's time to take another stab at adding healthy habits to your life, first take an honest look at what went wrong. If the habit didn't take because you made excuses, it might be as easy as restarting the same challenge with renewed resolve. Google "Shia LaBeouf Just Do It," and get back in the saddle. If you couldn't stick with it because you were attempting unrealistic changes, it's time to rethink the process and reevaluate your

# 7 DAY HEALTH CHALLENGES
## FOR WHEN YOU NEED A KICK IN THE ASS

*While there's no such thing as a quick fix, sometimes a jump start can be just what you need to get headed in the right direction. If you need a reason to start making changes, grab a friend and pick a challenge.*

| | | |
|---|---|---|
| **WATER** | Drink a gallon of water (128 oz) | Water can have an impact on your eating choices, stress levels, energy while exercising, and quality of sleep. This is a relatively easy challenge to commit to, and is particularly helpful when you feel like *everything* is out of control. |
| **SQUATS** | Start on day one with a number of squat repetitions and increase by a set amount (between five and ten reps) each subsequent day | This is a perfect one to do in your pajamas as soon as you get out of bed in the morning. It'll help you wake up, and push you in the right direction with your exercise goals. |
| **SLEEP** | Get five cycles each night by going to bed at the same time and waking up at the same time - weekends count! | This challenge will get your body on a schedule that is both consistent and sufficient in regards to your sleep needs. Even if you don't keep it up, it should help you recover from any recent shortcomings with sleep. This is a great one to do with your roommate. |
| **DESSERT** | No dessert after meals | By scrapping dessert from your diet for a week, you will come face-to-face with your sugar cravings. Being mindful about your consumption of sweets is hard because they're so easy to access, but doing a reset will hopefully allow you to reintroduce dessert on your own terms. |
| **BOOZE** | No drinking | It can be helpful to give yourself a reset with booze, particularly when you feel like you've been going out too often or drinking quite a lot. You can pair this with the sleep challenge to really give your body a chance to heal itself, or go out anyway and be the DD and drink soda water and limes for the night. |
| **STRETCHING** | Free stretch for fifteen minutes each day | This may end up feeling more like meditation than exercise, and that's OK. Give yourself some time to stretch without the pressure of an agenda while listening to music or a podcast. This "you time" can be valuable in helping manage your stress. |
| **SCHEDULE** | Write out a schedule for the next day each night before you to go to bed | Taking time at night to organize yourself for the coming day is a great way to download any stress from your brain before you go to sleep. Schedule in time to work out and study so that you end each day feeling even better about how much ass you kicked. |

*A challenge ups the ante when you want to make changes with your health. Don't feel restricted to the ones above. Consider any area of your health that is suffering and create your own challenge. Adding something positive to your life is typically easier than taking something away, but frankly, you can do anything for a week. Seven days of repeating a behavior isn't nearly long enough for it to become a habit, but if you notice a difference in your body or attitude as a result of the challenge, consider extending your commitment.*

expectations. Maybe working out three times a day and living off phytoplankton supersmoothies was a bad idea? Remember, taking care of yourself is a long-term thing—one you'll be chipping away at for the rest of your life. It's more sustainable to adopt relatively easy healthy behaviors one at a time then it is to dive headfirst into a slew of drastic changes that will be too hard to uphold. You may last a few weeks, but at some point the system will break.

It's also possible that in some way, the habit you want to form clashes with your identity.[29] If you've always been someone who eats the entire pizza or keeps the party going way into the night, then setting the intention to eat better, drink less, or sleep more may contradict how others see you. *After all, you don't get a nickname like "the Wolfman" for nothing.* People often underestimate what a hurdle this kind of clash can be. If you find yourself here, talk about your goals with a supportive friend who loves you for more than your ability to shotgun beers in quick succession. Don't compromise on your health goals because you're afraid of how other people are going to take it or see you. You've got to put your needs ahead of their judgment. And frankly, if your friends are shitting on your desire to be healthier and happier, maybe you should find new friends! Or be an example to them of what it looks like to make mature decisions. There are a whole lot of people in this world. Don't attach yourself to anchors that will just drag you down.

## For When You Forget

Because at some point, you're going to stop taking care of yourself and will wind up feeling like shit. When you're ready to clean it up, start here:

- **Identify the Area of Need.** You won't start feeling better if you can't figure out why you feel terrible. Food. Booze. Exercise. Stress. Sleep. Which areas of your health have been neglected? Once you've identified the component that feels most unstable, dive in, and figure out which microbehaviors seem to be causing problems by asking yourself follow-up questions. What is causing you to guzzle sugar, get to bed later than you want to, stress too much, bail on your workouts, or drink more than you know you should?

It's empowering to simply face what's been making you feel lousy and begin the process of game-planning a solution.

- **Introduce a Habit.** Habits take care of decision making for us, so by adopting habits that get us to make decisions that are good for our health, we reduce the effort required to stay healthy. Determine the specifics of the positive behavior you want to introduce, and know which cue will jump-start it. If you're able to keep a routine going long enough, it will become ingrained in your day, making it impervious to excuses and able to unfold without thought. This is how you will find yourself getting healthier and healthier over time and deviating less often.

- **Stick with It.** It's not easy to hold on to good behaviors, so prepare yourself with solutions to strengthen your resolve. Plan breaks, build in accountability, consider convenience, and learn to adjust when life gets in the way of your routine. The longer you hold on to a habit, the more likely it is to stick, and the easier it will be to come back to it when you stray.

Try to remember:

- **Start Over. Again.** If you're committed to taking care of yourself for the rest of your life, prepare to spend a lot of time getting off track, starting over, and then getting off track again. For those who are healthy, the work never stops. In fact, the thing that separates those who are healthy from those who aren't is a willingness to keep putting effort into it. If you never quit on yourself, then you never actually fail. You're ready.

# GRADUATION

**I've always been a planner.** As an eight-year-old, I created a scale model of my bedroom and made cutouts for each piece of furniture so I could test the feasibility of different layouts to decide on the best one before moving any of my stuff. When I went to my first sleepaway summer camp at twelve, I typed up a packing list with bullets for the individual items of clothing I was bringing, so I'd have something to cross-reference before leaving to ensure that nothing was left behind. I also used to eat Play-Doh and draw penis doodles in window dust, so don't be too impressed.

As someone who took comfort in having a plan, my first few weeks at college were both exciting and overwhelming. I realized that I could go out whenever I wanted to. Head to bed whenever I wanted to. Wake up whenever I wanted to. It began to sink in that every decision was mine to make, from short-term ones, such as what to eat, when to study, and whether or not to work out, to big-picture ones, such as the overwhelming question of what to *do* with my life. I believed it was my responsibility to know all the answers, so I dealt with the difficult uncertainties of college by solely focusing on my future.

I was already "over" college as a junior and only got less interested in being part of the scene as graduation neared. I couldn't stop thinking about being an "adult," and student teaching off-campus during my senior year further contributed to my preoccupation with what was coming next. At the time, I was living with my two best friends, one of whom regularly reminded me how much I was missing by not

223

living in the moment. She spent our final semester squeezing satisfaction and happiness out of each day. While I was working on my résumé, she was out on the quad playing Frisbee. While I was filling out job applications and researching the best cities to live in, she was lounging in a kiddie pool that she'd set up in our living room. I was busy obsessing over the vision board I'd created for my future, while she was enjoying the present. She'd like you to know, by the way, that she turned out to be a fully functioning adult as well.

That said, I enjoyed dreaming about the future. I always found comfort in the image that I had crafted of my adult life. It was *perfect*. How could it not be? People don't dream of failure, struggle, and redirection. That's only stuff you experience when you live in the present. It's much easier to think about what *could* be rather than what is, so why not spend time in that space? I had no reason not to. It wasn't clear to me until much later that my future was dependent on my present.

Only after dealing with a lot of frustration and unhappiness did I eventually shift my focus from the question "what does the future look like?" to "what does today look like?" The difference it made was unreal. It caused me to stumble upon a version of daily life that I was completely and truly satisfied with. One that, it turned out, I actually had a whole lot more control over. It just so happens that the little things you do for yourself every single day end up dictating who you are and where you're headed much more than a fascination with the future does.

We have control over many of our choices, but particularly those that determine our well-being. Health is the very foundation that holds us up and keeps us going day in and day out, and the stronger that foundation, the more confident and capable we are in everything that we do. Those dreams you have? Those goals you keep thinking about? Keep them! Make plans. Dream huge. But realize that you'll get where you want to be much faster if you focus on how to take care of yourself right now. And all the shit that is inevitably going to get in your way? You'll be better equipped to deal with it when coming from a place of inner strength.

The pyramid on the next page is "Maslow's Hierarchy of Needs," which you might recognize if you've taken a Psych 101 class. Maslow believed that everyone has an innate desire to reach their full potential and crush at life. He also believed that everyone has needs, and they must fulfill a series of basic ones before they can

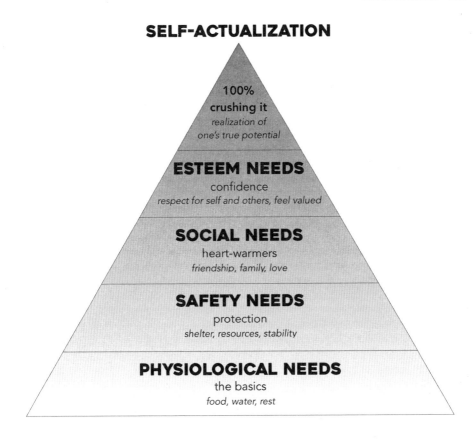

# SELF-ACTUALIZATION

**100%
crushing it**
*realization of
one's true potential*

## ESTEEM NEEDS
confidence
*respect for self and others, feel valued*

## SOCIAL NEEDS
heart-warmers
*friendship, family, love*

## SAFETY NEEDS
protection
*shelter, resources, stability*

## PHYSIOLOGICAL NEEDS
the basics
*food, water, rest*

move onward and upward toward becoming the best possible version of themselves, known as self-actualization.

Though it wasn't explicitly designed with health in mind, it's not a stretch to make that leap. The very bottom of the pyramid—the foundation—represents basic body needs: food, water, and rest. Expand rest to include stress management and exercise, and lump booze in with food, and it quickly comprises all the areas we need to manage to be healthy. You can't climb the pyramid if you don't have the foundation locked down, which implies that health is fundamentally important if we want to dominate in life.

However, feeling unstoppable is as fleeting as being healthy *because* they're connected. You may experience periods of complete self-assurance, but that doesn't mean you're going to stay there indefinitely. Your ability to continue crushing it tomorrow is dependent on how you care for your body and mind today. The more effort you put into keeping a solid base, the longer you'll be able to hang out on the rooftop deck with a smile on your face, wholly satisfied with your current situation but also wildly excited for your future. If you stop putting effort into your health, it'll only be a matter of time before you're back on the ground floor dreaming about what that "perfect" life is supposed to look like.

But you know what? You will stop putting effort into your health at some point. I guarantee it. No one is infallible. You're going to "fail" in plenty of areas where you'd rather not, and your health is going to be one of them. But instead of ignoring the state you're in or acknowledging it only to then feel terrible about yourself, I encourage you to accept it shamelessly. Living in the present requires the ability to recognize the existence of failure and know how to reframe it so it's useful moving forward. Which doesn't involve hiding under a blanket of your own guilt and disappointment. Burn *that* fucking blanket! Find a way to be proud of who you are and applaud yourself for having the desire to do better. That desire alone makes you special. It's a powerful motivator, and it's not held by everyone. But *you* have it. You have to. Otherwise, you would never have made it through a book like this. So give yourself props when you make a good choice rather than denigrating yourself when you make a bad one. Own the life you're living, and if you don't like it, *do something about it*. If you enjoy making plans, then keep most of them short-term and primarily consider how specific actions will make you *feel* physically and mentally immediately afterward.

We all spend time *not* living our "best life." After all, the top of that self-actualization pyramid is slippery. It's easy to tumble back down to the bottom. It's to be expected. But it's also possible to get your feet back under you and reach the top again, and it gets easier every time. With experience, you'll have a better idea of how to restart with your health, and every time you get going again, you'll be strengthened by the confidence of having done it before. Plus, now that you have a baseline understanding of the different domains of health, you can capitalize on the fact that they work together. Research suggests that mastering one area of your health positively impacts the others.[1] When you're eating well, it's easier to exercise.

Once you're exercising, it's easier to sleep. Eating well doesn't *cause* exercise, but it seems to make the introduction of it less painful. Who wants to go for a run with a belly full of beer, burgers, and fries? In essence, making improvements with any one area of your health is likely to have a spillover effect that reduces the effort required to make changes in other areas. You know the areas now. Pick a place to start and get moving. Only good things will follow.

Everything up until college can feel like traveling on a narrow trail. Guardrails and obstacles box you in from both sides, providing a pretty unambiguous path. And then one day, the trail opens into a field—a large flower-filled, mountain-framed pasture of grass that looks utterly spectacular from the edge. Full of endless routes and possibilities. That's life, and it starts with college for many people. The future is so vast that it can be overwhelming at times, mainly because there are no signposts or blazes, just a general sense of "this way." Sure, there are trees and other paths on the far side where the trail will pick up again, and the direction will be obvious, but it's not completely clear where or when that's going to happen. So stop worrying about that right now. When you're feeling unsure or lost or frustrated or scared, let good health be your compass. It'll always get you headed in the right direction. Enjoy your journey.

## PART 2: DAVE

**I always thought I needed to *be* something.** A doctor. A lawyer. A *something*. I felt the pressure of "what do you want to be when you grow up" from an early age, both from the outside world and my inner voice. The truth is, I never really knew. I tried on different majors and pictured myself in multiple professions, but I couldn't clearly see a dream job or a career path that felt like the right fit. Part of the problem was that I was focusing on what I wanted *to be* instead of focusing on what I wanted *to do*. *Being* something seemed so far away, like an impossible destination, I wouldn't be reaching any time soon. *Doing* something was easier to wrap my mind around, because it broke down the abstract *something*, a doctor, into a simple action, helping people. Full disclaimer, I'm not a doctor, but this method of breaking down broad, complicated goals into small, manageable actions forever changed my life.

In the summer after my freshman year, I had reached a point where I was tired of the way I was living, and I wanted to make a change. Not just with my health, but as a person in general, I wanted to be better. But what does that even look like? *Being* better. Everything boiled down to my behavior. We are a summation of our daily actions. So the only way for me to change into who I wanted to be was to change the things I was regularly doing. And the first step to making any changes was a thorough personal assessment. A comprehensive check-in with myself, like an accountant analyzing how you spend your money, made me focus on how I was spending my time. How much sleep did I get last night? The night before? What did I eat yesterday? When was the last time I worked out? How much time did I spend on my phone? Once I got the hang of where I needed to look, exploring all these categories eventually was replaced by asking myself one simple question: *How am I doing?* And for this internal assessment to have a real impact on my life, I had to be completely honest with myself. Which was really scary at first. The desire to only show the world the best parts of me and the tendency to gloss over the rough edges was an easy trap to fall into. It took making a lot of mistakes and painting myself into a corner before it finally hit me like a ton of bricks: I wanted to be better, and it was more important to me to move in *that* direction than it was to continue walking the path I'd been on. And holy shit, it was so freeing to finally put all that judgment down, look myself in the mirror, and begin a conversation that was based in truth.

I encourage you to start this dialogue with yourself, periodically checking in and doing so in the most honest way possible. This type of reflection is good for your soul. You are the only expert on your life, and your full testimony is required to make any changes. It might not be easy, as sometimes you're going to find things you're not proud of. Other times, you'll be so distracted with your day-to-day obligations, you'll simply forget to do it. But I can't stress enough how important it is to take a look at yourself in the mirror and be honest with the person you see. For me, the key to making significant positive changes has always begun with finding little places to improve. And now you have a whole book full of those small places to start with! Be kind to yourself. No matter what that voice in your head might say at times, you are worth it, and you can do it.

Beyond taking a look at *what you do*, consider *whom* you're doing it with. The people we surround ourselves with have a tremendous impact on our health, so when you check in for your internal assessment, take a look at your external group. Some people provide support and accountability. Others dish out discouragement or distraction. You deserve to be around people who are positive forces in your life, so be picky with who makes the cut. A pretty incredible research project called the Harvard Study of Adult Development started with the goal of answering the question, "What makes people healthy and happy?" The most startling revelation, according to study director Robert Waldinger, is that our relationships and how happy we are in them have a powerful influence on our health. Close relationships, more than money or fame, are what keep people happy throughout their lives.[2] And being happy keeps us healthy. Quality connections provide warmth in our hearts and protect us from life's curveballs. We actually feel less pain when things are painful and more joy when things are going our way. So don't settle! Move on from friends who make you feel bad about yourself and don't date vampire assholes who suck the life out of you. Instead, spend some time and energy in college taking care of yourself *and* building up your network of great people. Investing in quality relationships will pay enormous dividends, and I can't emphasize enough the importance of doing that in person.

It might be easier to follow or add a friend, but take the leap to see if someone will meet you for coffee, go for a walk, or just hang out anywhere. Have face-to-face interactions, ask questions, *listen*, and allow others to share about themselves with you. If you effectively respect and support someone, it makes them feel good. You can literally change someone's mood all because you listened and made them feel heard. There are good people everywhere, and by practicing giving people respect and attention, you'll inevitably stumble into some real human connections. Those are the real connections that will keep you happy long after the joy from getting a good grade in that hard class or nabbing that prestigious internship has faded. In the meantime, be grateful for any of the people currently in your life who make you feel supported and loved—parent, friend, coach, professor—whoever it might be.

Let them know they're great and that you love them back, and you'll see that it feels just as good to deliver kindness as it does to receive it.

Your health and your relationships will impact your future, and your future starts now. It's *your* turn. College marks the beginning of the rest of *your* life! So begin by establishing a set of basic rules that you're going to live by. Rules about how you spend your time, who you hang out with, and what your relationship is going to be with food, booze, exercise, stress, and sleep. Be honest about where you need to put in work, but talk kindly to yourself in the process, and try not to compare your progress to everyone else's. It never helps.

Remember that you will never be perfect, and there will be times when you stop trying altogether. There will be plenty of things grabbing at your attention and energy, and your health and happiness will, at some point, take a back seat as a result. That's okay. All you have to do is take note and start again. The payoff is always worth the effort, and this book will be here to remind you how to get going again if (or when) you need a refresher.

If you haven't found your big open field of possibility yet, you will soon. You may be excited, or you may be terrified, but what really matters is that it's time to move forward. We wrote this book to help you get through that field and to the other side. We're not giving you an *exact* path to follow; you must determine what works for you. The beauty of independence lies in the mystery of exploration. However, it helps to have a general sense of direction so you can avoid the thorn bushes, gopher holes, and steep cliffs. *Who puts cliffs in a field?!* We hope we've provided you with just enough guidance that your trip across is safe and smooth, but still full of choice and adventure. May you land on the other side feeling strong, confident, happy, and with a solid foundation in place for the future that lies ahead. Have some laughs, lock down some good habits, try not to shit your pants, and, most importantly, take care of yourself out there. We're rooting for you.

# ACKNOWLEDGMENTS

**We vividly remember the moment the idea for this project came into being.** We were excited, but also intimidated, by the prospect of working together on something for an audience that means so much to us both. If we were going to do it, we wanted to do it right. Ultimately, it was the unwavering optimism and support of our very own team that gave us the courage to push forward.

This book is dedicated to the cross-country girls—it would not exist without you. From the bottom of our hearts, thank you. It is an enormous privilege to be included in your lives, and we are constantly inspired by witnessing your grit, growth, and capacity. You and your families have been a steady source of support for us as we've grown together and started a family of our own. You've provided us with more love, joy, and purpose than you can imagine.

It was always important to us to include student voices, but we never dreamed we'd receive so many thoughtful responses. We'd like to extend an enormous thank-you to the many college students who participated in our survey. We know that spring semester free time is precious and can't adequately express how much we appreciate you writing in detail about your experiences so that we could share them here. Your stories are honest, open, raw, and hilarious. It was a privilege to get a glimpse into your world.

To our favorite math and psychology power couple, Vince Mateus and Monika Lind. You were the first people whose brains we picked about this project, and the final draft benefited enormously from the two days we all spent in Oregon talking for hours about the content that should be featured. We always gain perspective and knowledge from conversations with you both, and we're grateful for our many years of friendship.

We are honored that several health professionals were willing to lend their time and expertise to review of our work. Eric LeClair, Monika Lind, Allison Warren, Carrie Motschwiller, and Jesse Barglow: your thoughtful feedback helped us fine-tune each chapter and gave us confidence that we'd approached these topics in considerate and valuable way. Thank you so much.

We begged many friends and family to read an early (and, in retrospect, quite rough) version of this book to help us make it better. Lilly Maxfield, Natalie Rose Schwartz, Pete Riehl, and Connor Matthews, thank you for making time to get through and give feedback on a 220-page Word document while simultaneously balancing work and many other responsibilities. Your insight as students and recent graduates was invaluable. Kelly Mullane: from the get-go, you've believed in our ability to do this. You said that when we decided we were going to write a book, you knew it was going to happen. Your confidence in us, interest in this project, and support the whole way through kept us motivated when it started to feel overwhelming. We have benefited tremendously from your wisdom and life experience. Thank you for always offering us honest, uncensored feedback and for being one of the most important people in both our lives. Connie and Bob Henry, Janet Riehl, Bill and Lisa Riehl, and Mariana Riehl, thank you for believing in us now and always, for enthusiastically reviewing drafts, and for being genuinely invested in this collaboration of ours. We feel so lucky to have spent our whole lives with you on our team. Thank you for pointing us in the right direction and teaching us the importance of putting in the work, while also giving us the freedom to make mistakes.

We are fortunate to have people in our lives who simply have better taste than we do. We leaned heavily on Crista Flanagan, Alexei Dmitriew, Paul Cross, Jamie Martin, Jacob and Jessica Lane, Haley Buntrock, Ben Code, William Mason, Ani Pridjian, Lori Pridjian, Caroline Wresin, Sasha Codiga, Hope Codiga, Molly Schwartz, Lauren Montes, Katherine Montes, Haley Allen, Guy and Cathy Henry, Mindi Miller, and Rob Henry to give us advice on everything from marketing, fonts, and cover designs to the actual title itself. Thank you so much for your thoughtful feedback. Frankly, we're shocked that all of you haven't blocked our numbers yet.

Ed Jordan and Helen Lavely, this shout-out feels like the least we can do after you graciously offered us your home in Ashland as the location for our very first writers' retreat. The earliest words written for this book were typed at your kitchen island while Mac learned to crawl on your floors. We'll never forget that special and exciting time in our lives. We'll never forget the view. We'll also never forget being hunted by a flock of enormous wild turkeys. Terrifying.

Writing a book together while trying to keep our infant alive *actually* required a village. To Ava Ferry, Molly Schwartz, Sinclaire Ledahl, and Caroline Wreszin, who entertained our son morning, noon, and night, weekend after weekend, while we retreated to coffee shops and offices to brainstorm, write, and argue in peace. This book never would have crossed the finish line without the love and care that you provided our little man. It is always hard to step away from time with him, but knowing how much he loved being with all of you made it easier to focus on the work that needed to get done.

We've believed in this project from day one, but still can't quite comprehend how far it's come since the initial giddy conversations we had about it while brushing our teeth at night. To Sandy Goroff, thank you for being the first person with publishing experience to look at our concept and truly convince us that it was worthy of a large audience. We never would have ended up here without your encouragement. To our wonderful agent, Lucy Cleland. It still feels wild to say that we have an *agent*. Thank you for believing in two coaches who had only ever written for fun. You warmly opened the door to the literary world and escorted us in. You share our passion for this project and have never lost faith in its potential. You've collaborated with us, pushed us, and championed us as authors. Developing a relationship with you has been one of the greatest joys of the publishing process. To our illustrator, Spahic Dinara, your graphics single-handedly elevated this book. Thank you for working with us to bring our vision to life. Another thank-you to Emir Oručević for inspiring the cover. We explored a lot of options, but always felt drawn to your original. And finally, thank you to our editor, Leah Zarra, for taking a chance on us. You polished our work but kept our voice intact and have honored our vision since the beginning. You made our dream a reality and didn't ask us to change our style in the process. We feel very fortunate to have ended up with you at Skyhorse.

Lastly, we have to thank our two favorite teammates—our kids, Mac and Cammie. We started this project seven months after Mac was born, and if all goes according to plan, it will be published when Cammie is six months old. This book feels like our baby too, but we'll never be as proud of it as we already are of you both.

# ENDNOTES

## Chapter 1: Orientation

1.  Heidi J. Wengreen and Cara Moncur, "Change in Diet, Physical Activity, and Body Weight among Young-Adults during the Transition from High School to College," *Nutrition Journal* 8, no. 1 (December 2009): 32, https://doi.org/10.1186/1475-2891-8-32.
2.  Phillip B. Sparling, "Obesity on Campus," *Preventing Chronic Disease* 4, no. 3 (July 2007): A72.

## Chapter 2: Food

1.  Alexandra G. DiFeliceantonio et al., "Supra-Additive Effects of Combining Fat and Carbohydrate on Food Reward," *Cell Metabolism* 28, no. 1 (July 2018): 33-44.e3, https://doi.org/10.1016/j.cmet.2018.05.018.
2.  "CDC Press Releases," CDC, January 1, 2016, https://www.cdc.gov/media/releases/2017/p1116-fruit-vegetable-consumption.html.
3.  David Benton and Hayley A. Young, "Reducing Calorie Intake May Not Help You Lose Body Weight," *Perspectives on Psychological Science* 12, no. 5 (September 2017): 703–14, https://doi.org/10.1177/1745691617690878.
4.  "Undergraduate Student Reference Group: Executive Summary: Spring 2019," accessed December 3, 2019, https://www.acha.org/documents/ncha/NCHA-II_SPRING_2019_UNDER GRADUATE_REFERENCE%20_GROUP_EXECUTIVE_SUMMARY.pdf.
5.  Institute of Medicine (US) Committee on Examination of Front-of-Package Nutrition Rating Systems and Symbols et al., *History of Nutrition Labeling* (Washington, DC: National Academies Press, 2010), https://www.ncbi.nlm.nih.gov/books/NBK209859/.
6.  OEHHA Admin, "The Proposition 65 List," OEHHA, https://oehha.ca.gov/proposition-65/proposition-65-list.
7.  Badreldin H. Ali et al., "Potassium Bromate–Induced Kidney Damage in Rats and the Effect of Gum Acacia Thereon," *American Journal of Translational Research* 10, no. 1 (January 15, 2018): 126–37.
8.  Carol Potera, "Diet and Nutrition: The Artificial Food Dye Blues," *Environmental Health Perspectives* 118, no. 10 (October 2010): A428.

9.   "Dietary Guidelines for Americans, Eighth Edition: Cut Down on Added Sugars," *Department of Health and Human Services*, March 2016, 2.

10.  Robert H. Lustig, Laura A. Schmidt, and Claire D. Brindis, "The Toxic Truth about Sugar," *Nature* 482, no. 7383 (February 2012): 27–29, https://doi.org/10.1038/482027a.

11.  Shu Wen Ng, Meghan M. Slining, and Barry M. Popkin, "Use of Caloric and Non-Caloric Sweeteners in US Consumer Packaged Foods, 2005–2009," *Journal of the Academy of Nutrition and Dietetics* 112, no. 11 (November 2012): 1828–1834.e6, https://doi.org/10.1016/j.jand.2012.07.009.

12.  Jennifer A. Nettleton et al., "Diet Soda Intake and Risk of Incident Metabolic Syndrome and Type 2 Diabetes in the Multi-Ethnic Study of Atherosclerosis (MESA)," *Diabetes Care* 32, no. 4 (April 1, 2009): 688–94, https://doi.org/10.2337/dc08-1799.

13.  "Hidden in Plain Sight," SugarScience.UCSF.edu, https://sugarscience.ucsf.edu/hidden-in-plain-sight/.

14.  Samadi, David, "Sugar Is Not Only a Drug but a Poison Too," HuffPost, January 6, 2016, https://www.huffpost.com/entry/sugar-is-not-only-a-drug-but-a-poison-oo_b_8918630.

15.  Anna Schaefer and Kareem Yasin, "Experts Agree: Sugar Might Be as Addictive as Cocaine," Healthline, accessed November 25, 2019, https://www.healthline.com/health/food-nutrition/experts-is-sugar-addictive-drug.

16.  Wilhelm Hofmann et al., "Everyday Temptations: An Experience Sampling Study of Desire, Conflict, and Self-Control," *Journal of Personality and Social Psychology* 102, no. 6 (June 2012): 1318–35, https://doi.org/10.1037/a0026545.

17.  Barry M. Popkin, Kristen E. D'Anci, and Irwin H. Rosenberg, "Water, Hydration and Health," *Nutrition Reviews* 68, no. 8 (August 2010): 439–58, https://doi.org/10.1111/j.1753-4887.2010.00304.x.

18.  Allison Aubrey and Maria Godoy, "75 Percent of Americans Say They Eat Healthy—Despite Evidence to the Contrary," NPR.org, accessed November 25, 2019, https://www.npr.org/sections/thesalt/2016/08/03/487640479/75-percent-of-americans-say-they-eat-healthy-despite-evidence-to-the-contrary.

19.  "Overweight & Obesity Statistics," National Institute of Diabetes and Digestive and Kidney Diseases, accessed January 29, 2020, https://www.niddk.nih.gov/health-information/health-statistics/overweight-obesity.

20.  Alice A. Gibson et al., "Accuracy of Hands v. Household Measures as Portion Size Estimation Aids," *Journal of Nutritional Science* 5 (July 11, 2016), https://doi.org/10.1017/jns.2016.22.

21.  Rae Jacobson, "Eating Disorders and College," Child Mind Institute, accessed November 25, 2019, https://childmind.org/article/eating-disorders-and-college/.

22.  Jacobson.

23.  "Eating Disorders on the College Campus" (National Eating Disorders Association, February 2013). http://www.nationaleatingdisorders.org/sites/default/files/CollegeSurvey/CollegiateSurveyProject.pdf.

24.  "Eating Disorders on the College Campus."

25.  "Eating Disorders on the College Campus."

26.  "Eating Disorders," National Institute of Mental Health, accessed February 13, 2020, https://www.nimh.nih.gov/health/topics/eating-disorders/index.shtml#part_145414.

## Chapter 3: Booze

1.  "Undergraduate Student Reference Group: Executive Summary: Spring 2019," accessed December 9, 2019, https://www.acha.org/documents/ncha/NCHA-II_SPRING_2019 _UNDERGRADUATE_REFERENCE%20_GROUP_EXECUTIVE_SUMMARY.pdf.

2.  Henry Wechsler and Toben F. Nelson, "What We Have Learned from the Harvard School of Public Health College Alcohol Study: Focusing Attention on College Student Alcohol Consumption and the Environmental Conditions That Promote It," *Journal of Studies on Alcohol and Drugs* 69, no. 4 (July 2008): 481–90, https://doi.org/10.15288/jsad.2008.69.481.

3.  Brian Borsari and Kate B. Carey, "Peer Influences on College Drinking: A Review of the Research," *Journal of Substance Abuse* 13, no. 4 (December 1, 2001): 391–424, https://doi .org/10.1016/S0899-3289(01)00098-0.

4.  Peter LeViness et al., "The Association for University and College Counseling Center Directors Annual Survey 2018," n.d., 75. aucccd.org/assets/documents/Survey/2018%20aucccd%20sur vey-public-revised.pdf.

5.  "Undergraduate Student Reference Group: Executive Summary: Spring 2019."

6.  "Undergraduate Student Reference Group: Executive Summary: Spring 2019."

7.  Hamin Lee, Sungwon Roh, and Dai Jin Kim, "Alcohol-Induced Blackout," *International Journal of Environmental Research and Public Health* 6, no. 11 (November 2009): 2783–92, https://doi .org/10.3390/ijerph6112783.

8.  Suzanne C. Swan et al., "Just a Dare or Unaware? Outcomes and Motives of Drugging ('Drink Spiking') among Students at Three College Campuses," *Psychology of Violence* 7, no. 2 (2017): 253–64, https://doi.org/10.1037/vio0000060.

9.  Kurt M. Dubowski, PhD, "Stages of Acute Alcoholic Influence/Intoxication" (Oklahoma City: University of Oklahoma, 2006), http://www.drugdetection.net/PDF%20documents /Dubowski%20-%20stages%20of%20alcohol%20effects.pdf.

10. "Understanding the Dangers of Alcohol Overdose," National Institute on Alcohol Abuse and Alcoholism (NIAAA), accessed April 25, 2019, https://www.niaaa.nih.gov/publications /brochures-and-fact-sheets/understanding-dangers-of-alcohol-overdose.

11. Dubowski, "Stages of Acute Alcoholic Influence/Intoxication."

12. Dubowski.

13. Dubowski.

14. M. Frezza et al., "High Blood Alcohol Levels in Women: The Role of Decreased Gastric Alcohol Dehydrogenase Activity and First-Pass Metabolism," *New England Journal of Medicine* 322, no. 2 (January 11, 1990): 95–99, https://doi.org/10.1056/NEJM199001113220205.

15. Martin S. Mumenthaler et al., "Gender Differences in Moderate Drinking Effects," *Alcohol Research & Health* 23, no. 1 (1999): 55–64.

16. Alex Paton, "Alcohol in the Body," *BMJ: British Medical Journal* 330, no. 7482 (January 8, 2005): 85–87.

17. Ron Weathermon, "Alcohol and Medication Interactions," *Alcohol Research & Health* 23, no. 1 (1999): 15.

18. "Micro RNA Implicated as Molecular Factor in Alcohol Tolerance," National Institute on Alcohol Abuse and Alcoholism (NIAAA), last modified July 30, 2008, https://www

.niaaa.nih.gov/news-events/news-releases/micro-rna-implicated-molecular-factor-alcohol
-tolerance.

19. "Fall Semester—A Time for Parents to Discuss the Risks of College Drinking," National Institute on Alcohol Abuse and Alcoholism (NIAAA), accessed April 25, 2019, https://www.niaaa .nih.gov/publications/brochures-and-fact-sheets/time-for-parents-discuss-risks-college-drinking.

20. Ralph Hingson et al., "Magnitude of Alcohol-Related Mortality and Morbidity Among U.S. College Students Ages 18–24: Changes from 1998 to 2001," *Annual Review of Public Health* 26, no. 1 (2005): 259–79, https://doi.org/10.1146/annurev.publhealth.26.021304.144652.

21. Wechsler and Nelson, "What We Have Learned from the Harvard School of Public Health College Alcohol Study."

22. U.S. Department of Transportation, "Time of Day and Demographic Perspective of Fatal Alcohol-Impaired-Driving Crashes," *National Highway Traffic Safety Administration*, August 2011, 8.

23. Harvard School of Public Health College Alcohol Study, "Binge Drinking on American College Campuses: A New Look at an Old Problem," last modified August 1995, http://archive.sph .harvard.edu/cas/rpt1994/CAS1994rpt2.html.

24. "About Bradley | B.R.A.D.," accessed November 26, 2019, http://brad21.org/about-bradley.

25. Elizabeth E. Lloyd-Richardson et al., "The Relationship between Alcohol Use, Eating Habits and Weight Change in College Freshmen," *Eating Behaviors* 9, no. 4 (December 2008): 504–8, https://doi.org/10.1016/j.eatbeh.2008.06.005.

26. Riccardo Vecchio, Azzurra Annunziata, and Angela Mariani, "Is More Better? Insights on Consumers' Preferences for Nutritional Information on Wine Labelling," *Nutrients* 10, no. 11 (November 4, 2018), https://doi.org/10.3390/nu10111667.

27. Robert Swift, "Alcohol Hangover," *Research World* 22, no. 1 (1998): 7.

28. Murray Epstein, "Alcohol's Impact on Kidney Function," *Research World* 21, no. 1 (1997): 10.

29. Arif Kadri Balcı et al., "General Characteristics of Patients with Electrolyte Imbalance Admitted to Emergency Department," *World Journal of Emergency Medicine* 4, no. 2 (2013): 113–16, https://doi.org/10.5847/wjem.j.issn.1920-8642.2013.02.005

30. Jeff Wiese et al., "Effect of Opuntia Ficus Indica on Symptoms of the Alcohol Hangover," *Archives of Internal Medicine* 164, no. 12 (June 28, 2004): 1334–40, https://doi.org/10.1001 /archinte.164.12.1334.

31. Tsukamoto S. et al., "Effects of Amino Acids on Acute Alcohol Intoxication in Mice— Concentrations of Ethanol, Acetaldehyde, Acetate and Acetone in Blood and Tissues," *Arukoru Kenkyu to Yakubutsu Izon = Japanese Journal of Alcohol Studies & Drug Dependence* 25, no. 5 (October 1, 1990): 429–40.

32. T. Seppälä et al., "Effects of Hangover on Psychomotor Skills Related to Driving: Modification by Fructose and Glucose," *Acta Pharmacologica et Toxicologica* 38, no. 3 (1976): 209–18, https: //doi.org/10.1111/j.1600-0773.1976.tb03113.x.

33. Swift, "Alcohol Hangover."

34. Arthur I. Cederbaum, "Alcohol Metabolism," *Clinics in Liver Disease* 16, no. 4 (November 2012): 667–85, https://doi.org/10.1016/j.cld.2012.08.002.

35. Hank Nuwer, "Hazing Deaths Database: Unofficial Hazing Clearinghouse & Watchdog Site," accessed November 27, 2019, http://www.hanknuwer.com/hazing-deaths/.

36. "Hazing Deaths on American College Campuses Remain Far Too Common," *Economist*, accessed February 2, 2020, https://www.economist.com/graphic-detail/2017/10/13/hazing-deaths-on -american-college-campuses-remain-far-too-common.

37. Harvard School of Public Health College Alcohol Study, "Binge Drinking on American College Campuses: A New Look at an Old Problem."

38. Harvard School of Public Health College Alcohol Study.

39. Sean Esteban McCabe, Philip Veliz, and John E. Schulenberg, "How Collegiate Fraternity and Sorority Involvement Relates to Substance Use During Young Adulthood and Substance Use Disorders in Early Midlife: A National Longitudinal Study," *Journal of Adolescent Health* 62, no. 3 (March 1, 2018): S35–43, https://doi.org/10.1016/j.jadohealth.2017.09.029.

40. Hingson et al., "Magnitude of Alcohol-Related Mortality and Morbidity Among U.S. College Students Ages 18–24."

41. Wechsler and Nelson, "What We Have Learned from the Harvard School of Public Health College Alcohol Study."

42. Harvard School of Public Health College Alcohol Study, "Binge Drinking on American College Campuses: A New Look at an Old Problem."

43. Ralph W. Hingson, Wenxing Zha, and Elissa R. Weitzman, "Magnitude of and Trends in Alcohol-Related Mortality and Morbidity among U.S. College Students Ages 18–24, 1998– 2005," *Journal of Studies on Alcohol and Drugs: Supplement*, no. 16 (July 2009): 12–20.

44. Bonnie S. Fisher, Francis T. Cullen, and Michael G. Turner, "The Sexual Victimization of College Women," *US Department of Justice*, Research Report, December 2000, 47.

45. Michael Planty, "Campus Climate Survey Validation Study Final Technical Report," n.d., 218.

46. Antonia Abbey, "Alcohol and Sexual Violence Perpetration," *National Online Resource Center on Violence Against Women*, 2008, 17.

47. Meichun Mohler-Kuo et al., "Correlates of Rape While Intoxicated in a National Sample of College Women," *Journal of Studies on Alcohol* 65, no. 1 (January 2004): 37–45, https://doi .org/10.15288/jsa.2004.65.37.

48. Brian A. Reaves, "Campus Law Enforcement, 2011–2012," *US Department of Justice*, January 2015, 27.

49. Michelle C. Black et al., "National Intimate Partner and Sexual Violence Survey: 2010 Summary Report," *National Center for Injury Prevention and Control, Centers for Disease Control and Prevention.*, 2010, 124.

50. Harvard School of Public Health College Alcohol Study, "Binge Drinking on American College Campuses: A New Look at an Old Problem."

51. "What Is Consent?," Sexual Assault Prevention and Awareness Center: University of Michigan, accessed November 27, 2019, https://sapac.umich.edu/article/49.

52. Kate B. Carey et al., "Precollege Predictors of Incapacitated Rape among Female Students in Their First Year of College," *Journal of Studies on Alcohol and Drugs* 76, no. 6 (November 2015): 829–37, https://doi.org/10.15288/jsad.2015.76.829.

53. "1 in 3 American Women Has Experienced Some Type of Sexual Violence," womenshealth. gov, accessed February 2, 2019, https://www.womenshealth.gov/relationships-and-safety /sexual-assault-and-rape/sexual-assault.

54. Reaves, "Campus Law Enforcement, 2011–2012."

55. "Know Your Rights on Campus: Sexual Harassment and Sexual Assault under Title IX," *American Association of University Women (AAUW): Empowering Women Since 1881* (blog), accessed November 27, 2019, https://www.aauw.org/what-we-do/legal-resources/know-your -rights-on-campus/campus-sexual-assault/.

56. "College Drinking," National Institute on Alcohol Abuse and Alcoholism (NIAAA), accessed April 25, 2019, https://www.niaaa.nih.gov/publications/brochures-and-fact -sheets/college-drinking.

57. "Treatment for Alcohol Problems: Finding and Getting Help," National Institute on Alcohol Abuse and Alcoholism (NIAAA), accessed April 25, 2019, https://www.niaaa.nih.gov /publications/brochures-and-fact-sheets/treatment-alcohol-problems-finding-and-getting-help.

58. "Alcohol Use Disorder," National Institute on Alcohol Abuse and Alcoholism (NIAAA), accessed February 2, 2019, https://www.niaaa.nih.gov/alcohol-health/overview-alcohol -consumption/alcohol-use-disorders.

59. "Alcohol Use Disorder," Psychology Today, accessed February 2, 2020, https://www.psychology -today.com/conditions/alcohol-use-disorder.

## Chapter 4: Exercise

1. "Exercise Survey Statistics in the US: Americans' Affinity with Sports," *Reportlinker Insight* (blog), May 31, 2017, https://www.reportlinker.com/insight/shape-americans-exercise-get-fit.html.

2. Debra L. Blackwell and Tainya C. Clarke, "State Variation in Meeting the 2008 Federal Guidelines for Both Aerobic and Muscle-Strengthening Activities Through Leisure-Time Physical Activity Among Adults Aged 18-64," *National Health Statistics Reports,* no. 112 (June 2018): 22.

3. "Summary: 2008 Physical Activity Guidelines: Health.Gov," accessed November 30, 2019, https://health.gov/paguidelines/2008/summary.aspx.

4. Sarah Elizabeth Linke, Linda C. Gallo, and Gregory J. Norman, "Attrition and Adherence Rates of Sustained vs. Intermittent Exercise Interventions," *Annals of Behavioral Medicine: A Publication of the Society of Behavioral Medicine* 42, no. 2 (October 2011): 197–209, https: //doi.org/10.1007/s12160-011-9279-8.

5. Lindsay R. Duncan et al., "Exercise Motivation: A Cross-Sectional Analysis Examining Its Relationships with Frequency, Intensity, and Duration of Exercise," *International Journal of Behavioral Nutrition and Physical Activity* 7 (January 26, 2010): 7, https://doi.org/10.1186/1479 -5868-7-7.

6. David Garner, "Body Image in America: Survey Results," Psychology Today, last reviewed September 14, 2017, http://www.psychologytoday.com/articles/199702/body-image-in-america -survey-results.

7. Darren E. R. Warburton, Crystal Whitney Nicol, and Shannon S. D. Bredin, "Health Benefits of Physical Activity: The Evidence," *CMAJ: Canadian Medical Association Journal* 174, no. 6 (March 14, 2006): 801–9, https://doi.org/10.1503/cmaj.051351.

8. "Exercise and Immunity: MedlinePlus Medical Encyclopedia," accessed November 30, 2019, https://medlineplus.gov/ency/article/007165.htm.

9. Li Yanping et al., "Impact of Healthy Lifestyle Factors on Life Expectancies in the US Population," *Circulation* 138, no. 4 (July 24, 2018): 345–55, https://doi.org/10.1161 /CIRCULATIONAHA.117.032047.

10. Mora Samia et al., "Physical Activity and Reduced Risk of Cardiovascular Events," *Circulation* 116, no. 19 (November 6, 2007): 2110–18, https://doi.org/10.1161/CIRCULATIONAHA .107.729939.

11. "Physical Activity and Cancer," National Cancer Institute, last reviewed February 10, 2020, https://www.cancer.gov/about-cancer/causes-prevention/risk/obesity/physical-activity-fact-sheet.

12. Rachel Hosie, "Is It Impossible to Change Your Personality Past the Age of 30?," *Independent*, June 14, 2017, http://www.independent.co.uk/life-style/personality-change-past-age-30-is-it -possible-psychology-kirsten-godfrey-david-buss-carol-rothwell-a7757866.html.

13. Jennifer Cohen, "6 Ways Exercise Makes You Smarter," Forbes, accessed December 2, 2019, https://www.forbes.com/sites/jennifercohen/2012/05/08/6-ways-exercise-makes-you-smarter/.

14. Christina DesMarais, "15 Daily Habits Highly Successful People Have (and the Rest of Us Probably Don't)," Inc.com, May 18, 2018, https://www.inc.com/christina-desmarais/15-daily -habits-highly-successful-people-have-and-rest-of-us-probably-dont.html.

15. Theresa E. DiDonato, "5 Reasons Why Couples Who Sweat Together, Stay Together," Psychology Today, accessed December 2, 2019, http://www.psychologytoday.com/blog/meet -catch-and-keep/201401/5-reasons-why-couples-who-sweat-together-stay-together.

16. Hamdi Chtourou and Nizar Souissi, "The Effect of Training at a Specific Time of Day: A Review," *Journal of Strength & Conditioning Research* 26, no. 7 (July 2012): 1984–2005, https: //doi.org/10.1519/JSC.0b013e31825770a7.

17. Chrisanna Northrup, "'Not Enough Time to Exercise' Is Just an Excuse," Huffpost, accessed December 2, 2019, https://www.huffpost.com/entry/exercise-excuse-internet_b_927097.

18. "Workout Worries," Fit Rated, accessed December 2, 2019, https://www.fitrated.com/resources /workout-worries/#fair-use-statement.

19. Matthew Cocks et al., "Sprint Interval and Endurance Training Are Equally Effective in Increasing Muscle Microvascular Density and ENOS Content in Sedentary Males," *Journal of Physiology* 591, no. Pt 3 (February 1, 2013): 641–56, https://doi.org/10.1113/jphysiol.2012.239566.

20. "Can You Boost Your Metabolism?," Mayo Clinic, accessed December 2, 2019, https: //www.mayoclinic.org/healthy-lifestyle/weight-loss/in-depth/metabolism/art-20046508.

21. "Hot Weather Running Tips," Road Runners Club of America, accessed January 30, 2020, https://www.rrca.org/education/hot-weather-running-tips.

22. Erin Beresini, "Why You Should Never, Ever Stop Training," Outside Online, March 29, 2016, https://www.outsideonline.com/2065496/science-behind-falling-out-shape.

## Chapter 5: Stress

1. "Adrenaline," You and Your Hormones, accessed December 3, 2019, https://www.yourhormones .info/hormones/adrenaline/.

2. "Chronic Stress Puts Your Health at Risk," Mayo Clinic, accessed December 3, 2019, https: //www.mayoclinic.org/healthy-lifestyle/stress-management/in-depth/stress/art-20046037.

3. "Undergraduate Student Reference Group: Executive Summary: Spring 2019," accessed December 3, 2019, https://www.acha.org/documents/ncha/NCHA-II_SPRING_2019_UNDER GRADUATE_REFERENCE%20_GROUP_EXECUTIVE_SUMMARY.pdf.

4. "Undergraduate Student Reference Group: Executive Summary: Spring 2019."

5.  Gina Shaw, "Water and Stress Reduction: Sipping Stress Away," WebMD, accessed December 3, 2019, https://www.webmd.com/diet/features/water-stress-reduction.

6.  Emma Childs and Harriet de Wit, "Regular Exercise Is Associated with Emotional Resilience to Acute Stress in Healthy Adults," *Frontiers in Physiology* 5 (2014), https://doi.org/10.3389/fphys.2014.00161.

7.  "Socialization and Altruistic Acts as Stress Relief," MentalHelp.net, accessed December 4, 2019, https://www.mentalhelp.net/stress/socialization-and-altruistic-acts-as-stress-relief/.

8.  Mary P. Bennett et al., "The Effect of Mirthful Laughter on Stress and Natural Killer Cell Activity," *Alternative Therapies in Health and Medicine* 9, no. 2 (April 2003): 38–45.

9.  Samira S. Bamuhair et al., "Sources of Stress and Coping Strategies among Undergraduate Medical Students Enrolled in a Problem-Based Learning Curriculum," *Journal of Biomedical Education*, 2015, https://www.hindawi.com/journals/jbe/2015/575139/.

10. Clifton B. Parker, "Embracing Stress Is More Important Than Reducing Stress, Stanford Psychologist Says," Stanford News, May 7, 2015, https://news.stanford.edu/2015/05/07/stress-embrace-mcgonigal-050715/.

11. James W. Pennebaker, Janice K. Kiecolt-Glaser, and Ronald Glaser, "Disclosure of Traumas and Immune Function: Health Implications for Psychotherapy," *Journal of Consulting and Clinical Psychology* 56, no. 2 (1998): 7.

12. Irina Sangeorzan, Panoraia Andriopoulou, and Maria Livanou, "Exploring the Experiences of People Vlogging about Severe Mental Illness on YouTube: An Interpretative Phenomenological Analysis," *Journal of Affective Disorders* 246 (March 1, 2019): 422–28, https://doi.org/10.1016/j.jad.2018.12.119.

13. Robert A. Emmons and Michael E. McCullough, "Counting Blessings versus Burdens: An Experimental Investigation of Gratitude and Subjective Well-Being in Daily Life," *Journal of Personality and Social Psychology* 84, no. 2 (February 2003): 377–89, https://doi.org/10.1037//0022-3514.84.2.377.

14. Kristin Layous et al., "The Proximal Experience of Gratitude," *PLoS ONE* 12, no. 7 (July 7, 2017), https://doi.org/10.1371/journal.pone.0179123.

15. Robert A. Emmons and Robin Stern, "Gratitude as a Psychotherapeutic Intervention: Gratitude," *Journal of Clinical Psychology* 69, no. 8 (August 2013): 846–55, https://doi.org/10.1002/jclp.22020.

16. "Undergraduate Student Reference Group: Executive Summary: Spring 2019."

17. Pablo Valdez, "Circadian Rhythms in Attention," *Yale Journal of Biology and Medicine* 92, no. 1 (March 25, 2019): 81–92.

18. Nathaniel Kleitman, "Basic Rest-Activity Cycle—22 Years Later," *Sleep* 5, no. 4 (September 1, 1982): 311–17, https://doi.org/10.1093/sleep/5.4.311.

19. Nathaniel Kleitman, *Sleep and Wakefulness*, Midway Reprint (Chicago: University of Chicago Press, 1987).

20. Kleitman.

21. Mihaly Csikszentmihalyi, *Flow* (New York: Harper Perennial Modern Classics, 2008).

22. David J. Shernoff et al., "Student Engagement as a Function of Environmental Complexity in High School Classrooms," *Learning and Instruction*, Special Issue: Student Engagement and Learning: Theoretical and Methodological Advances, 43 (June 1, 2016): 52–60, https://doi.org/10.1016/j.learninstruc.2015.12.003.

23. Norman B. Anderson et al., *Paying with Our Health* (Washington, DC: American Psychological Association, 2015).

24. Samantha Fields, "70% of College Students Graduate with Debt. How Did We Get Here?," *Marketplace* (blog), September 30, 2019, https://www.marketplace.org/2019/09/30/70-of-college-students-graduate-with-debt-how-did-we-get-here/.

25. "College Student Employment," National Center for Education Statistics, *The Condition of Education* 2019 (2019): 4.

26. "Dealing with Financial Stress," American Psychological Association, accessed January 30, 2020, https://www.apa.org/helpcenter/holiday-stress-finances.

27. Daniel Zapp, *2019 Money Matters Report* (AIG Retirement Services, 2019).

28. "Undergraduate Student Reference Group: Executive Summary: Spring 2019."

29. Nagesh Tumkur Subbarao and A. Akhilesh, "Knowledge and Attitude about Sexually Transmitted Infections Other than HIV among College Students," *Indian Journal of Sexually Transmitted Diseases and AIDS* 38, no. 1 (2017): 10–14, https://doi.org/10.4103/2589-0557.196888.

30. "Fast Facts About HPV," American Sexual Health Association, accessed February 12, 2020, http://www.ashasexualhealth.org/stdsstis/hpv/fast-facts/.

31. Adam Felman, "Stress: Why Does It Happen and How Can We Manage It?," Medical News Today, November 2017, https://www.medicalnewstoday.com/articles/145855.php.

32. Aaron Kandola, "Chronic Stress: Symptoms, Health Effects, and How to Manage It," Medical News Today, October 2018, https://www.medicalnewstoday.com/articles/323324.php.

33. "Undergraduate Student Reference Group: Executive Summary: Spring 2019."

34. Ben Locke, "2018 Annual Report" (Center for Collegiate Mental Health, January 2019), https://ccmh.psu.edu/files/2019/09/2018-Annual-Report-9.27.19-FINAL.pdf.

35. "Undergraduate Student Reference Group: Executive Summary: Spring 2019."

36. "Depression Basics," National Institute of Mental Health, accessed December 5, 2019, https://www.nimh.nih.gov/health/publications/depression/index.shtml.

37. Chanrith Ngin et al., "Social and Behavioural Factors Associated with Depressive Symptoms among University Students in Cambodia: A Cross-Sectional Study," *BMJ Open* 8, no. 9 (September 28, 2018), https://doi.org/10.1136/bmjopen-2017-019918.

38. "Depression: What You Need to Know," National Institute of Mental Health, accessed December 6, 2019, https://www.nimh.nih.gov/health/publications/depression-what-you-need-to-know/index.shtml.

39. LeViness et al., "The Association for University and College Counseling Center Directors Annual Survey 2018."

40. "Undergraduate Student Reference Group: Executive Summary: Spring 2019."

41. James C. Turner, E. Victor Leno, and Adrienne Keller, "Causes of Mortality among American College Students: A Pilot Study," *Journal of College Student Psychotherapy* 27, no. 1 (January 1, 2013): 31–42, https://doi.org/10.1080/87568225.2013.739022.

42. Holly C. Wilcox et al., "Prevalence and Predictors of Persistent Suicide Ideation, Plans, and Attempts during College," *Journal of Affective Disorders* 127, no. 1–3 (December 2010): 287–94, https://doi.org/10.1016/j.jad.2010.04.017.

43. Anemona Hartocollis, "His College Knew of His Despair. His Parents Didn't, Until It Was Too Late," *New York Times*, May 12, 2018, sec. U.S., https://www.nytimes.com/2018/05/12/us/college-student-suicide-hamilton.html.

44. Daniel Eisenberg et al., "Mental Health Service Utilization among College Students in the United States," *The Journal of Nervous and Mental Disease* 199, no. 5 (May 2011): 301–8, https://doi.org/10.1097/NMD.0b013e3182175123.

## Chapter 6: Sleep

1. Mark R. Zielinski, James T. McKenna, and Robert W. McCarley, "Functions and Mechanisms of Sleep," *AIMS Neuroscience* 3, no. 1 (2016): 67–104, https://doi.org/10.3934/Neuroscience.2016.1.67.
2. Zielinski, McKenna, and McCarley.
3. "Undergraduate Student Reference Group: Executive Summary: Spring 2019."
4. A. G. Wheaton et al., "Short Sleep Duration among Middle School and High School Students—United States, 2015," *MMWR: Morbidity and Mortality Weekly Report* 67 (2018): 85–90, https://doi.org/10.15585/mmwr.mm6703a1.
5. "Undergraduate Student Reference Group: Executive Summary: Spring 2019."
6. Luciana Besedovsky, Tanja Lange, and Jan Born, "Sleep and Immune Function," *Pflugers Archiv* 463, no. 1 (January 2012): 121–37, https://doi.org/10.1007/s00424-011-1044-0.
7. Matthew D. Milewski et al., "Chronic Lack of Sleep Is Associated with Increased Sports Injuries in Adolescent Athletes," *Journal of Pediatric Orthopedics* 34, no. 2 (March 2014): 129–33, https://doi.org/10.1097/BPO.0000000000000151.
8. Rachel Leproult and Eve Van Cauter, "Role of Sleep and Sleep Loss in Hormonal Release and Metabolism," in *Endocrine Development*, ed. S. Loche et al., vol. 17 (Basel: KARGER, 2009), 11–21, https://doi.org/10.1159/000262524.
9. Michele Bellesi et al., "Sleep Loss Promotes Astrocytic Phagocytosis and Microglial Activation in Mouse Cerebral Cortex," *Journal of Neuroscience* 37, no. 21 (May 24, 2017): 5263–73, https://doi.org/10.1523/JNEUROSCI.3981-16.2017.
10. Bellesi et al.
11. "Sleep and Mental Health," Harvard Health, accessed December 11, 2019, https://www.health.harvard.edu/newsletter_article/sleep-and-mental-health.
12. "Stress and Sleep," American Psychological Association, accessed December 10, 2019, https://www.apa.org/news/press/releases/stress/2013/sleep.
13. "Sleep and Mental Health."
14. Shelley D. Hershner and Ronald D. Chervin, "Causes and Consequences of Sleepiness among College Students," *Nature and Science of Sleep* 6 (June 23, 2014): 73–84, https://doi.org/10.2147/NSS.S62907.
15. William Edward Kelly, Kathryn E. Kelly, and Robert Clanton, "The Relationship between Sleep Length and Grade-Point Average among College Students," vol. 35 (College Student Journal, 2001), 84–88.
16. Mark R. Rosekind et al., "Alertness Management: Strategic Naps in Operational Settings," *Journal of Sleep Research* 4, no. s2 (1995): 62–66, https://doi.org/10.1111/j.1365-2869.1995.tb00229.x.
17. "What Happens during Sleep?," Eunice Kennedy Shriver National Institute of Child Health and Human Development, accessed December 11, 2019, https://www.nichd.nih.gov/health/topics/sleep/conditioninfo/what-happens.

18. "What Happens during Sleep?"
19. "Brain Basics: Understanding Sleep," National Institute of Neurological Disorders and Stroke, accessed December 11, 2019, https://www.ninds.nih.gov/Disorders/Patient-Caregiver-Education/Understanding-Sleep#2.
20. "What Happens during Sleep?"
21. "Brain Basics: Understanding Sleep."
22. M. H. Hagenauer et al., "Adolescent Changes in the Homeostatic and Circadian Regulation of Sleep," *Developmental Neuroscience* 31, no. 4 (June 2009): 276–84, https://doi.org/10.1159/000216538.
23. Hagenauer et al.
24. Nick Littlehales, *Sleep: The Myth of 8 Hours, the Power of Naps, and the New Plan to Recharge Your Body and Mind* (New York: Da Capo Lifelong Books, 2018).
25. Littlehales.
26. Hans P. A. Van Dongen et al., "The Cumulative Cost of Additional Wakefulness: Dose-Response Effects on Neurobehavioral Functions and Sleep Physiology from Chronic Sleep Restriction and Total Sleep Deprivation," *Sleep* 26, no. 2 (March 15, 2003): 117–26, https://doi.org/10.1093/sleep/26.2.117.
27. Maggie Jones, "How Little Sleep Can You Get Away With?," *New York Times*, April 15, 2011, sec. Magazine, https://www.nytimes.com/2011/04/17/magazine/mag-17Sleep-t.html.
28. Mitsuo Hayashi, Akiko Masuda, and Tadao Hori, "The Alerting Effects of Caffeine, Bright Light and Face Washing after a Short Daytime Nap," *Clinical Neurophysiology* 114, no. 12 (December 1, 2003): 2268–78, https://doi.org/10.1016/S1388-2457(03)00255-4.
29. Jiunn-Horng Kang and Shih-Ching Chen, "Effects of an Irregular Bedtime Schedule on Sleep Quality, Daytime Sleepiness, and Fatigue among University Students in Taiwan," *BMC Public Health* 9 (July 19, 2009): 248, https://doi.org/10.1186/1471-2458-9-248.
30. Kang and Chen.
31. Littlehales, *Sleep: The Myth of 8 Hours, the Power of Naps, and the New Plan to Recharge Your Body and Mind.*
32. Kostadin Kushlev and Elizabeth W. Dunn, "Checking Email Less Frequently Reduces Stress," *Computers in Human Behavior* 43 (February 1, 2015): 220–28, https://doi.org/10.1016/j.chb.2014.11.005.
33. Popkin, D'Anci, and Rosenberg, "Water, Hydration and Health."
34. "Extent and Health Consequences of Chronic Sleep Loss and Sleep Disorders," in *Sleep Disorders and Sleep Deprivation*, ed. H. R. Colten and B. M. Altevogt (Washington, DC: National Academies Press, 2006), https://www.ncbi.nlm.nih.gov/books/NBK19961/.
35. "Sleep Deprivation," Columbia University Department of Neurology, accessed February 2, 2020, http://www.columbianeurology.org/neurology/staywell/document.php?id=42069.
36. Hannah G. Lund et al., "Sleep Patterns and Predictors of Disturbed Sleep in a Large Population of College Students," *Journal of Adolescent Health: Official Publication of the Society for Adolescent Medicine* 46, no. 2 (February 2010): 124–32, https://doi.org/10.1016/j.jadohealth.2009.06.016.
37. A. Williamson and A. Feyer, "Moderate Sleep Deprivation Produces Impairments in Cognitive and Motor Performance Equivalent to Legally Prescribed Levels of Alcohol Intoxication,"

*Occupational and Environmental Medicine* 57, no. 10 (October 2000): 649–55, https://doi .org/10.1136/oem.57.10.649.

38. Flavie Waters et al., "Severe Sleep Deprivation Causes Hallucinations and a Gradual Progression Toward Psychosis with Increasing Time Awake," *Frontiers in Psychiatry* 9 (July 10, 2018), https: //doi.org/10.3389/fpsyt.2018.00303.

39. Caroline R. Mahoney et al., "Intake of Caffeine from All Sources and Reasons for Use by College Students," *Clinical Nutrition* 38, no. 2 (April 1, 2019): 668–75, https://doi.org/10.1016/j .clnu.2018.04.004.

40. Marla Rivera-Oliver and Manuel Díaz-Ríos, "Using Caffeine and Other Adenosine Receptor Antagonists and Agonists as Therapeutic Tools against Neurodegenerative Diseases: A Review," *Life Sciences* 101, no. 1–2 (April 17, 2014): 1–9, https://doi.org/10.1016/j.lfs.2014.01.083.

41. Christopher Drake et al., "Caffeine Effects on Sleep Taken 0, 3, or 6 Hours before Going to Bed," *Journal of Clinical Sleep Medicine* 9, no. 11 (November 15, 2013): 1195–1200, https://doi .org/10.5664/jcsm.3170.

42. Timothy Roehrs and Thomas Roth, "Sleep, Sleepiness, and Alcohol Use," National Institute on Alcohol Abuse and Alcoholism, accessed December 11, 2019, https://pubs.niaaa.nih.gov /publications/arh25-2/101-109.htm.

43. Roehrs and Roth.

44. Steve Sussman et al., "Misuse of 'Study Drugs:' Prevalence, Consequences, and Implications for Policy," *Substance Abuse Treatment, Prevention, and Policy* 1 (June 9, 2006): 15, https://doi .org/10.1186/1747-597X-1-15.

45. Shankar Sadasivan et al., "Methylphenidate Exposure Induces Dopamine Neuron Loss and Activation of Microglia in the Basal Ganglia of Mice," *PLoS ONE* 7, no. 3 (March 21, 2012), https://doi.org/10.1371/journal.pone.0033693.

46. Gianluca Tosini, Ian Ferguson, and Kazuo Tsubota, "Effects of Blue Light on the Circadian System and Eye Physiology," *Molecular Vision* 22 (January 24, 2016): 61–72.

47. Jiexiu Zhao et al., "Red Light and the Sleep Quality and Endurance Performance of Chinese Female Basketball Players," *Journal of Athletic Training* 47, no. 6 (2012): 673–78.

48. Angelo Cagnacci et al., "Homeostatic versus Circadian Effects of Melatonin on Core Body Temperature in Humans," *Journal of Biological Rhythms* 12, no. 6 (December 1997): 509–17, https://doi.org/10.1177/074873049701200604.

49. Damien Leger et al., "Poor Sleep Is Highly Associated with House Dust Mite Allergic Rhinitis in Adults and Children," *Allergy, Asthma & Clinical Immunology* 13, no. 1 (August 16, 2017): 36, https://doi.org/10.1186/s13223-017-0208-7.

## Chapter 7: Trial and Error

1. Roma Pahwa, Anand Singh, and Ishwarlal Jialal, "Chronic Inflammation," in *StatPearls* (Treasure Island, FL: StatPearls Publishing, 2020), http://www.ncbi.nlm.nih.gov/books/NBK493173/.

2. Pahwa, Singh, and Jialal.

3. Ananda R. Ganguly and Joshua Tasoff, "Fantasy and Dread: The Demand for Information and the Consumption Utility of the Future," SSRN Scholarly Paper (Rochester, NY: Social Science Research Network, May 16, 2016), https://papers.ssrn.com/abstract=2370983.

4. James A. Roberts, Luc Honore Petnji Yaya, and Chris Manolis, "The Invisible Addiction: Cell-Phone Activities and Addiction among Male and Female College Students," *Journal of Behavioral Addictions* 3, no. 4 (December 2014): 254–65, https://doi.org/10.1556/JBA.3.2014.015.

5. "Time Flies: U.S. Adults Now Spend Nearly Half a Day Interacting with Media," Neilson, accessed December 12, 2019, https://www.nielsen.com/us/en/insights/article/2018/time-flies-us-adults-now-spend-nearly-half-a-day-interacting-with-media.

6. Roberts, Petnji Yaya, and Manolis, "The Invisible Addiction."

7. Roberts, Petnji Yaya, and Manolis.

8. Erik Peper and Richard Harvey, "Digital Addiction: Increased Loneliness, Anxiety, and Depression," *NeuroRegulation* 5, no. 1 (March 30, 2018): 3–3, https://doi.org/10.15540/nr.5.1.3.

9. Elliot Panek, "Left to Their Own Devices: College Students' 'Guilty Pleasure' Media Use and Time Management," *Communication Research* 41, no. 4 (June 1, 2014): 561–77, https://doi.org/10.1177/0093650213499657.

10. Barry R. Schlenker, Beth A. Pontari, and Andrew N. Christopher, "Excuses and Character: Personal and Social Implications of Excuses," *Personality and Social Psychology Review* 5, no. 1 (February 1, 2001): 15–32, https://doi.org/10.1207/S15327957PSPR0501_2.

11. Benjamin Gardner, Phillippa Lally, and Jane Wardle, "Making Health Habitual: The Psychology of 'Habit-Formation' and General Practice," *British Journal of General Practice* 62, no. 605 (December 2012): 664–66, https://doi.org/10.3399/bjgp12X659466.

12. Gardner, Lally, and Wardle.

13. Wendy Wood, Jeffrey M. Quinn, and Deborah Kashy, "Habits in Everyday Life: Thought, Emotion, and Action.," *Journal of Personality and Social Psychology* 83, no. 6 (2002): 1281–97, https://doi.org/10.1037//0022-3514.83.6.1281.

14. Charles Duhigg, *The Power of Habit: Why We Do What We Do in Life and Business* (New York: Random House, 2012).

15. James Clear, "The Habit Loop: 5 Habit Triggers That Make New Behaviors Stick," *James Clear* (blog), February 24, 2015, https://jamesclear.com/habit-triggers.

16. Marina Milyavskaya and Michael Inzlicht, "What's So Great About Self-Control? Examining the Importance of Effortful Self-Control and Temptation in Predicting Real-Life Depletion and Goal Attainment," *Social Psychological and Personality Science* 8, no. 6 (August 2017): 603–11, https://doi.org/10.1177/1948550616679237.

17. Nicholas A. Christakis and James H. Fowler, "The Spread of Obesity in a Large Social Network over 32 Years," *New England Journal of Medicine* 357, no. 4 (July 26, 2007): 370–79, https://doi.org/10.1056/NEJMsa066082.

18. Daniel Pink, *Drive: The Surprising Truth about What Motivates Us* (Riverhead Books, New York, NY, 2011).

19. T. W. Malone et al., "Toward a Theory of Intrinsically Motivating Instruction," 1981.

20. Mihaly Csikszentmihalyi, "Play and Intrinsic Rewards," in *Flow and the Foundations of Positive Psychology: The Collected Works of Mihaly Csikszentmihalyi*, ed. Mihaly Csikszentmihalyi (Dordrecht: Springer Netherlands, 2014), 135–53, https://doi.org/10.1007/978-94-017-9088-8_10.

21. Valarmathie Gopalan et al., "A Review of the Motivation Theories in Learning" (The 2nd International Conference on Applied Science and Technology 2017 [ICAST'17], Kedah, Malaysia, 2017), 020043, https://doi.org/10.1063/1.5005376.

22. Phillippa Lally et al., "How Are Habits Formed: Modelling Habit Formation in the Real World," *European Journal of Social Psychology* 40, no. 6 (2010): 998–1009, https://doi.org/10.1002/ejsp.674.

23. Gretchen Rubin, *Better Than Before: What I Learned about Making and Breaking Habits—to Sleep More, Quit Sugar, Procrastinate Less, and Generally Build a Happier Life* (New York: Broadway Books, 2015).

24. Joel Constable, "Two Techniques for Helping Employees Change Ingrained Habits," *Harvard Business Review*, March 28, 2018, https://hbr.org/2018/03/two-techniques-for-helping-employees -change-ingrained-habits.

25. Elias Oussedik et al., "Accountability: A Missing Construct in Models of Adherence Behavior and in Clinical Practice," *Patient Preference and Adherence* 11 (July 25, 2017): 1285–94, https://doi .org/10.2147/PPA.S135895.

26. "Low on Self-Control? Surrounding Yourself with Strong-Willed Friends May Help," Association for Psychological Science, accessed February 2, 2020, https://www.psychologicalscience.org /news/releases/low-on-self-control-surrounding-yourself-with-strong-willed-friends-may-help .html.

27. Michael L. Lowe and Kelly L. Haws, "(Im)Moral Support: The Social Outcomes of Parallel Self-Control Decisions," *Journal of Consumer Research* 41, no. 2 (August 1, 2014): 489–505, https://doi.org/10.1086/676688.

28. Peter M. Gollwitzer et al., "When Intentions Go Public: Does Social Reality Widen the Intention-Behavior Gap?," *Psychological Science* 20, no. 5 (May 1, 2009): 612–18, https://doi .org/10.1111/j.1467-9280.2009.02336.x.

29. "Finding It Hard to Change a Habit? Maybe This Explains Why," Gretchen Rubin, accessed February 2, 2020, http://gretchenrubin.com/2014/07/finding-it-hard-to-change -a-habit-maybe-this-explains-why/.

## Graduation

1. Benjamin Gardner, Phillippa Lally, and Jane Wardle, "Making Health Habitual: The Psychology of 'Habit-Formation' and General Practice," *British Journal of General Practice* 62, no. 605 (December 2012): 664, https://doi.org/10.3399/bjgp12X659466.

2. Liz Mineo, "Over Nearly 80 Years, Harvard Study Has Been Showing How to Live a Healthy and Happy Life," *Harvard Gazette* (blog), April 11, 2017, https://news.harvard.edu/gazette /story/2017/04/over-nearly-80-years-harvard-study-has-been-showing-how-to-live-a-healthy -and-happy-life/.

# INDEX